Dysmobility in Geriatrics

José Luis Dinamarca-Montecinos

Dysmobility in Geriatrics

Conceptualisation, Clinical Approach, and Aging Theory

Springer

José Luis Dinamarca-Montecinos
Orthogeriatric Program
Hospital Dr. Gustavo Fricke
Viña del Mar, Chile

ISBN 978-3-031-72715-3 ISBN 978-3-031-72716-0 (eBook)
https://doi.org/10.1007/978-3-031-72716-0

This Springer imprint is published by the registered company Springer Nature Switzerland AG
The registered company address is: Gewerbestrasse 11, 6330 Cham, Switzerland

Dedicated

to Perfect Movement,

to Infinity Love.

The Author

Foreword

This book is fruit of a professional persistence and commitment for advancing in our understanding of the essential keys of life and aging: that is the Movement-Time Theory, life and aging as the eternal product of movement and time. Individual and humankind life as a continuum of biological and physical movement over time, from the very initial developmental phase to advanced ages, from the Earth's birth to everyday individual births and deaths—both, milestones in the journey from the initial to the last breath of mobility, and examples of the transformative phases of the universal legacy.

Focusing on mobility changes, the Dysmobility approach represents a captivating and provocative framework for understanding the complexities of health and disease, to better define the medical answers and social services, needed for aging-related personal needs affecting the individual's ability to maintain independence and quality of life.

One could imagine human life, from the body's development phase up to the extremely advanced ages, as the combination of motions across environment and time to get resources for a quality survival and living. And the body's machinery sustaining homeostasis and leading to continuous internal movements, then interactions with the environment generating the main determinants of life, health, and quality of life.

Mobility, as the sum of individual movements experienced over time, will summarize intrinsic vitality, leading to different degrees of expression according to biological strata and interconnection levels of functioning, from micro to macro, in the body's structural and functional dynamics.

The body's ultimate strive of the dynamic movement is maintaining homeostasis through continuous interactions with the environment, which are pivotal for health and quality of life. Indeed, throughout life, humans adapt their movements to changing environmental conditions. For instance, adapting to seasonal changes by altering physical activity patterns or modifying living spaces to accommodate aging-related mobility issues.

Dysmobility abruptly or slowly can significantly affect individuals' homeostasis and health outcomes, promoting the acceleration of the entropy related forces at the individual and ecosystem levels.

Then, understanding the concept of Dysmobility not only proposes strategies to enhance care and mitigate human suffering while aging. It also provides significant insights when considering the aging process within the broader context of human evolution and ecosystem adaptation throughout the life course.

Integrating Dysmobility syndrome into healthcare systems underscores the importance of movement at every stage of life as a means to maintain health, quality of life, and resilience against disease, and to promote healthy aging.

By promoting healthy mobility, we can ultimately enhance individual well-being and societal health, and contribute to the sustainability of human life in our planet. It is likely the secret for counteracting or delaying the system's entropy at the individual, societal, and species levels.

This perspective aligns with the continuous dance of elements within our bodies, environments, and the broader ecosystem, emphasizing the interconnectedness of health and mobility in the entire universe.

Gerontology and Geriatric Section
Department of Medicine and Surgery
University of Perugia
Perugia, Italy

Orthogeriatric and Geriatric Acute Care Units
Perugia University Hospital
Perugia, Italy

The Fragility Fracture Network - Italia
Rome, Italy

Carmelinda Ruggiero

Prologue

The world is experiencing a significant demographic shift with falling birth rates and increasing life expectancy, placing age and aging at the centre stage of social, economic, political, health and academic debate.

José Luis Dinamarca, in this massive immersive experience—*Dysmobility in Geriatrics*—challenges the traditional view of the birth, life and death of individuals and how mobility and 'Dysmobility' is viewed by society. Here, we are presented with the idea that living beings begin to age 'before' existing and continue to age 'after' dying. *Dysmobility in Geriatrics* also encourages the reader to challenge assumptions about the connection between movement and time (Dysmobility Theory) and that chronological years lived does not explain *when* we age or *how* we age. In fact, aging generates, in parallel, two effects: deterioration and maturation—and one does not occur without the other. As we all move through time, we also develop skills, create links, complete achievements, generate knowledge and acquire wisdom, and these are not signs of deterioration.

This is a refreshing and optimistic view of aging in comparison to the perhaps too commonly held negative stereotypes which tend to be associated with deterioration, ill health, and decline.

This book presents age and aging within the context of the whole person *and* the universe in which they live. It will present you with big ideas, it will challenge assumptions and, most importantly, it will give you a practical toolkit to support your everyday clinical practice and assessment of the older person. I beckon you to dive straight into Chap. 1.

This is exactly what I did, and I was delighted, that as a Physiotherapist I was immediately challenged within the first few pages to re-frame my own perception of mobility and immobility. Instead, I now channel my thoughts within the context of Dysmobility.

One of the most important concepts presented in this book is that everything is moving continuously, movement does not pause. *'Even when sleeping, we can say that we execute a set of movements that allow us to rest'*. This seems obvious to me now that I have experienced the journey through *Dysmobility in Geriatrics*, but previously I had been trained to treat the person with immobility—and the physical and emotional consequences resulting from this.

José Luis Dinamarca guides readers like me gently through key stages, from considering human movement at a molecular level, the genetic level, and the system level (and the interdependent continuum "NEMOH": Neuro Endocrine Muscle Osseum Hematological) and then allowing them to place this in the context of Dysmobility as a geriatric syndrome.

Dysmobility, as a geriatric syndrome, consists of discomfort, difficulty and/or an inability to move part of the body, and this occurs secondary to various pathological situations which can be of *any* origin (biological, psychological, social, spiritual, functional, etc.). Dysmobility affects quality of life and/or can have a risk of progression. Throughout Chap. 4 the method of triaxial diagnosis of Dysmobility—the geriatric syndrome—is presented. We learn to define the presentation as slow or abrupt and then we can apply D-STAGING, a dynamic system consisting of 10 substages. We move deeper throughout Chap. 5 learning to integrate time and understand the concept of progression, which can move Dysmobility towards deeper stages, and stabilization and regression which can move Dysmobility towards earlier stages. The reader then moves towards the end of the book gaining practical assessment and diagnostic prompt cards (Chap. 6), the luxury of a full history of the evidence base of Dysmobility (Chap. 7), and example clinical cases (Chap. 8).

I therefore leave you now, with another delight and revelation to me—the paraphrase from Descartes '*I move therefore I am*' (Chap. 9). Dysmobility as a diagnosis and a concept allows us to place the person within their whole spiritual, societal, physical, and emotional context; movement is constantly present at all levels, and everything can be mediated through movement—which never stops—I move therefore I am.

Let us all go into the world, equipped with the knowledge presented in these pages, to make a difference to those we support and care for, and to make a difference to ourselves.

University of Birmingham
Birmingham, UK

Emma L. Sutton

University Hospitals Birmingham NHS Foundation Trust
Birmingham, UK

Preface

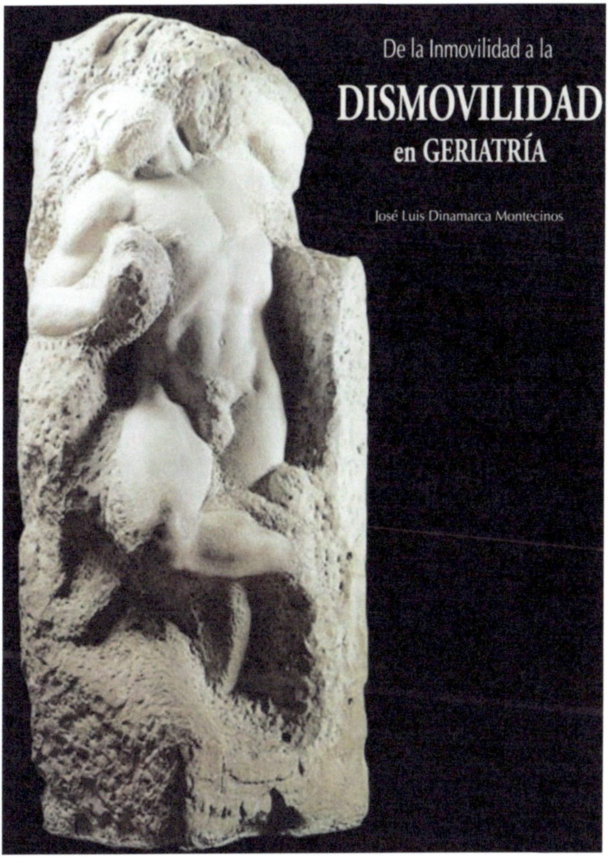

Fig. 1 Original frontcover of the first Spanish edition of the book "From Immobility to Dysmobility in Geriatrics" (SOCHIPSI Editions, Santiago de Chile 2004)

The year was 2001 and I was responsible for taking charge of the then-called 'Prostrate Program' of the Santo Tomás Hospital, in the city of Limache, in the region of Valparaíso, in Chile. The patients were mainly elderly people who couldn't get out of bed, but I also fondly remember a little girl and her mother who took care of her.

With a small group of professionals and technicians, we toured the city every Tuesday between 8 a.m. and 2 p.m. in a van, visiting the program's patients in their homes. Our resources were limited, so I had to limit our actions and responsibilities. As a result of several meetings, in the middle of the year we generated a regulation, which operated a set of guidance notes to improve management of this patient population.

Within the guidance, we divided the city into nine parts, conducting visits every 3 months, so that we could visit all our patients four times a year on a scheduled basis. I remember that we tried to define 'prostrate patient' without much success, even though we were reviewing the literature for several months.

In the end, we changed the name of the program, from 'prostrate program' to 'Home Care Program'. The eligibility criteria were summarized in the phrase 'any patient who, with the means available to him, cannot go to the nearest health centre when needed, due to permanent medical conditions'. There were other administrative and organizational criteria (for example, the city in which patients live) that helped us decide eligibility and who would be accepted on the program, mainly because we only had time and capacity for 63 people in that condition.

In December of the same year, I started working at the city's Geriatric specialty hospital, the La Paz de la Tarde Geriatric Hospital. In my enthusiasm for the work we had done throughout the year, I made it a condition to be able to allocate part of my hours to continue working in the Home Care Program. Dr. Ernesto Rojo Flores, Director of the Geriatric Hospital, a doctor with a lot of vision, must have been a little surprised by this request, but he backed my request and, in turn setting a condition, he asked me to send a summary of our work to the National Congress of the Society of Geriatrics and Gerontology of Chile, during October 2002. Without thinking about it (or perhaps, thinking about it) I had begun the search for a true clinical definition of Immobility syndrome. I had 10 months to achieve it.

During that time, I began studying a Diploma in Geriatrics at the University of Concepción, and several doors opened for me to understand geriatric semiology, pathophysiology, and epidemiology, especially through the study of Geriatric syndromes. I had come to the right place, and I came face to face with Immobility syndrome and Dr. Isaacs'i's': immobility, instability, intellectual impairment, incontinence, and iatrogenic complications. I knew what I was looking for, but the definitions of Immobility syndrome were not satisfactory for me, as they did not provide answers to our needs in the Home Care Program. They did nothing to support our eligibility criteria, they did not establish any relationship with the old word 'prostration' and, most frustratingly, they did not allow us to establish any management plan for our patients.

I began to consider whether the problem was that the syndrome was being approached from a static perspective: as the ***result*** of a process, rather than as a ***process with several stages***. 'Immobility' never seemed static me: even the most apparently immobile of our patients breathed, moved their eyes, their heart beats and, of course, although most of them could not be understood, we knew that they felt and perceived our care. Then, I could not accept limiting mobility to a purely locomotor issue. Our patients were not 'immobile…' I found that I had a question to answer: if our Home Program patients were not 'immobile', how were they?

The answer to this question arrived sooner than I thought: They are in the final stages of a set of motor problems, they are having motor difficulties, with problems moving around well. That is, our patients are experiencing DYS-mobility, not IM-mobility.

It was like a revelation. I ran to search for the term 'Dysmobility', but the Google entries from that time, almost 25 years ago, returned less than 10 results. Among them, however, the chapter 'Immobility and Dysmobility', from the book *Primary Care in Geriatrics: Clinical Cases* [1].

However, once I got the book, I didn't find any definition of Dysmobility in the corresponding chapter! The word only appeared in the title, and the entire chapter was dedicated to the well-known Immobility syndrome.

Other results in Spanish gave responses for 'Dysmotility', associating it with disorders in the motility of the cilia of respiratory cells in children [2]. The results in English also did not show any results for 'Dysmobility'.

I decided to start working on the topic with my Diploma teachers. Dr. Federico von Mühlembrock and Dr. Ernesto Rojo supported me enthusiastically, showing from the first moment that they were in favour of further work: an entire reconceptualization of the classic Immobility syndrome. I had to dedicate time to it, and I presented my early work at the IV Latin American Congress of Geriatrics and Gerontology organized by the Latin American Committee of the IAGG in Santiago de Chile, between September 3 and 6, 2003.

The title, which was accepted and published in the Congress abstract book, was: *Immobility Syndrome: Situational Diagnosis and Home Care Project*. Their acceptance was, however, a great incentive to continue focusing on our Home Program patients. One effect of this was a new proposed name for our home program: Home Care Program for Dysmobilized Patients (PADIS, for its acronym in Spanish). The name was accepted, and I began to work on our official clinical guidance notes, which was published during March 2004.

The objective of this guidance was to facilitate the work of my team and those who would come in the future, so that, in turn, patients could benefit more from their work. In the guidance I define the concepts of Dysmobility and dysmobilizing process, and I propose several stages in said process. I also proposed that if the diagnosis was narrowed enough, populations from various rehabilitation centres could be compared, to define the best therapeutic processes for each group of patients according to their stage.

We were very happy with those clinical guidance notes because we realized that they would help us enormously to better define progression and prognosis of our patients, better decide treatments, and to work with their caregivers, landing their expectations.

I clearly remember what happened next, so please allow me to give a small literary touch to this technical book:

The light did not make any effort to enter the doctors' room at the Geriatric Hospital, decisively illuminating the circular surface of the coffee table and making the glass that covered it shine. On top of it, I had placed five copies of the PADIS clinical guidance notes, freshly ringed and each with a smoke-coloured cover. They looked perfect, ready to be distributed to my team members, as a surprise, during the meeting that we would have in just 45 min. The shadow of a man obscured the light shining on the glass for a fleeting moment, and then transformed into a person: my friend Andrés Dadal.

- What are those booklets?

Andrés asked me in his pleasant lilting conversation.

I proudly explained, and I was quite surprised by how captivated Andrés was by my answer… At the end, they are just simple clinical guidance notes…

- It is not a simple clinical guidance...—He said—. It is a concept that deserves to be known by many others. Let me make a phone call.

And that's how, in a matter of minutes, I was in contact with the manager of Andrés' laboratory, Elías Chahuán. After a little conversation, I sent him one of the booklets containing our clinical guidance notes, and Elías's enthusiasm and support for the concept allowed us to transform those notes into the first book on Dysmobility. It was April 2004, and I registered a copy of the clinical guidance notes which I published as *Dysmobility in Geriatrics*, in my name, in the National Registry of Intellectual Property.

Subsequently, at the request of the enthusiastic Director of the Geriatric Hospital, Dr. Ernesto Rojo Flores, I sent three abstracts to the IX National Congress of the Society of Geriatrics and Gerontology of Chile, which that year was held in Viña del Mar. The abstracts had a huge impact among the attendees and the Scientific Committee, and they were proposed as winners of the Congress. I sent the expanded works to the Latin American Network of Gerontology (RLG, for its acronym in Spanish), because during the Congress I had met Ximena Romero, Sociologist and Coordinator of the Network, who had been very enthusiastic about the concept of Dysmobility. Thanks to her efforts, the works were posted on the RLG website during the first weeks of September 2005, announcing the launch of the book.

The book was called *From Immobility to Dysmobility in Geriatrics*. As its cover, it had *The Prisoners*, one of Michelangelo's unfinished sculptures for the tomb of Pope Julius II (Fig. 1). The book was published under the seal of the Chilean Society of Psychogeriatrics (SOCHIPSI, for its acronym in Spanish). The first (and only) edition of *From Immobility to Dysmobility in Geriatrics* printed 1000 copies, which were sold out in the following years.

The launch of *From Immobility to Dysmobility in Geriatrics* took place on September 30, 2005, in a surprisingly packed auditorium of the Limache Geriatric Hospital. It had media and even political impact: The launch was publicized prominently in the newspaper *El Observador* (from the cities of Limache, Quillota, and La Calera) [3], and a copy of the book was requested to be deposited in the Library of the National Congress, which was completed in January 2006.

Since then, entries for the word 'Dysmobility' on Google have continually increased, with different implications. The concept of Dysmobility and its methodology became used across the Spanish-speaking world, both in Latin America and in Spain, within some months.

Scientific works published in indexed journals that used the proposed classification began to appear, and the book was cited in several university graduate programs; and degree theses on the topic of Dysmobility were carried out for various health careers.

By 2008, I had directed my steps towards Granada, Spain, and I trained as a Doctor in Social Gerontology at the University of Granada. First, I applied for a Scholarship from the MAPFRE Foundation, seeking to give a higher level to the concept of Dysmobility, ensuring that the concept could relate to the origins of aging. Thus, in 2007 the project 'Theory of Dysmobility: Movement, time, and aging. In search of the bases of a single Theory of

Aging' (in Spanish: Teoría de la Dismovilidad. Movimiento, tiempo y envejecimiento. En búsqueda de las bases de una única Teoría del Envejecimiento), won a place among the Ignacio Hernando de Larramendi 2007 Research Grants [4]. This work became the main body of my research to qualify for the Diploma of Advanced Studies of the Doctorate in Social Gerontology at the University of Granada, in 2009.

In 2011, Dysmobility celebrated its first decade and we celebrated it with an article published in the Viña del Mar Hospital Bulletin in 2012 [5], which summarized many of the concepts that appeared in the out-of-print 2005 book.

By the time we reached two decades of the Dysmobility concept being in use in clinical and research settings, the COVID-19 pandemic had arrived, and an article to commemorate 20 years of the concept born in Limache was delayed. We began to work instead on a Portuguese translation for use in Brazil.

And then, during 2023, I was contacted by Springer to translate the Dysmobility concept into English. With this most recent English translation, I hope with all my heart that this book is useful to many, in many more decades to come.

Viña del Mar, Valparaíso, Chile José Luis Dinamarca-Montecinos

References

1. Murphy JB. Chapter 13: Dysmobility and immobility. In: Ham RJ, Sloane PD, editors. Primary care in geriatrics: clinical cases. Part 2. Mosby/Doyma; 1995. pp. 312–333.
2. Mur Sierra A, Viñolas Tolosa M, Sánchez García Vao C, García López AC, Busquets Monge RM, García Algar O, Lloreta Trull J, Bargués Cardelús R. Asociación entre el consumo de heroína durante la gestación y anomalías estructurales de los cilios respiratorios en el período neonatal. Anales Pediatría. 2001;55(4):335–8.
3. https://www.bibliotecanacionaldigital.gob.cl/bnd/628/w3-article-261607.html.
4. https://app.mapfre.com/ccm/content/documentos/fundacion/salud/becas/fallo-2007-becaslarramendi.pdf.
5. Dinamarca-Montecinos JL. Dysmobility in geriatrics. A decade defining a clinical concept. Bol Hosp Vina del Mar. 2012;68(2):15–9.

Acknowledgment

With contributions by

Emma L Sutton (PhD, MSc, BSc, HCPC)
External Reviewer and Reference for Conceptual Translation
Associate Professor, University of Birmingham, Birmingham, United Kingdom
Clinical Academic Lead (Nurses, Midwives, Allied Health Professionals) University Hospitals Birmingham NHS Foundation Trust, Birmingham, United Kingdom

Carmelinda Ruggiero (MD, PhD, MSc)
External Reviewer and Reference for Concepts in Geriatrics
Associate Professor, University of Perugia, Perugia, Italy
Director of the School of Specialisation in Geriatrics, Department of Medicine and Surgery, University of Perugia, Perugia, Italy
Head of the Orthogeriatric unit, Academic Hospital S Maria della Misericordia, Perugia, Italy
President, the Fragility Fracture Network, Italy

Cecilia Bonta Arias (MSc, BSc)
External Reviewer in Clinical Case in Logopedics
Special collaboration in the development of the Movement-Time Theory
Private clinical practice of Geriatric Logopedics

Soraya León Araya (PhD, MSc)
External Reviewer in Clinical Case in Geriatric Dentistry
Associated Professor, University of Talca, Talca, Chile
Director of the Graduate Program in Geriatric Dentistry, University of Talca, Talca, Chile
Coordinator, thematic line about Geriatric Dentistry, Interuniversity Centre for Healthy Aging (CIES), Consortium of State Universities of Chile (CUECH)

Viviana García Ubillo (MSc, BSc)
External Reviewer in Clinical Case in Logopedics
Associated Professor, University of Valparaíso, Valparaíso, Chile
Coordinator, Diploma in Gerontogeriatric Phonoaudiology, University of Valparaíso, Valparaíso, Chile
Director, Geropolis Centre, University of Valparaíso, Valparaíso, Chile
Coordinator, thematic line about Quality of Life and Social Determinants of Healthy Aging, Interuniversity Centre for Healthy Aging (CIES), Consortium of State Universities of Chile (CUECH)

Contents

Human Movement: What Is It?

1

Introduction

The main purpose of this book is to provide useful advice and guidance for everyday clinical practice, from a new conceptual perspective of movement, time, and aging.

While the book can be used by clinical staff working 'on the ground', some of the concepts presented could be challenging from an academic point of view, where the problems may be difficult to unravel or define. Therefore, the concepts which will be expressed in the first chapters will enable you to gain an initial approach to understand the concept of Dysmobility.

To fully immerse the reader in the concept of Dysmobility, this chapter will take the reader from practice to the conceptual world and then back again, so that practice can be evidence-informed.

What Is Movement? From One Definition to Another

A Physical Definition of Movement

Movement can be understood as the change in the position of a body, over time, with respect to a reference system [1]. The study of movement depends on physics and mechanics and, within it, kinematics, and dynamics. Seen this way, movement is a phenom-

J. L. Dinamarca-Montecinos, *Dysmobility in Geriatrics*, https://doi.org/10.1007/978-3-031-72716-0_1

enon of positional dynamics that occur in time. An important aspect of this definition is that movement *never* occurs 'alone': Necessarily, 'something' is moving, and that something is always a body.

We could (arbitrarily) vary the definition of 'physical body', leaving it just as 'body', and understand the concept of 'body' as 'any element that is subject to movement'. This would include physical ***and non-physical bodies***, which will be 'bodies' because they move, such as thoughts and more abstract concepts such as knowledge, emotions, and soul.

Another point of this definition that cannot go unnoticed is that a reference system is essential for the study of movement. This is because everything is moving continuously. The movement has no pause.

Let us digest that sentence again—***'movement has no pause'***.

This brings us to introduce the concept that immobility is just an illusion—it does not really exist. To fully explain it, we need to always think of using a reference point. For example, if we limit the movement of a rock to our immediate surroundings, it will appear to be completely still. However, if we broaden our reference to the planet, we will realise that even the most seemingly immobile of rocks is orbiting at incredible speed.

Likewise, on a biological scale, every cubic micron of cytoplasm, every pyrimidic base, is constantly moving. Even when sleeping, we can say that we execute a set of movements that allow us to rest. In fact, sleep is part of a stable cycle of motor routines, the sleep-wake cycle.

Now that we have introduced you to the idea that immobility does not exist, it may be possible to consider a clinical definition of movement as a continuous phenomenon.

A 'Clinical' Definition of Movement

Movement can be defined as follows: a continuous phenomenon, composed of the constant spatiotemporal changes made by a body/occurring in a body.

To use this definition, and allow the definition to be easily applied in practice, it is necessary to define some levels. This is necessary because the levels at which movement occurs are infinite, so they will depend on many factors, including the knowledge we have of our reality, and the taxonomy we use.

On a biological scale, we could progressively speak of molecular, genetic, chromosomal, cellular, tissue, and systemic movement. We will briefly refer to the first three to exemplify the perspective of the movement.

Movement at the Molecular Level

There are many molecules in our body. Some are known to everyone. Others are a bit cryptic, and only a few experts know about them. All of them are interrelated. Their functions intersect and are mutually dependent. In some cases, the genesis of some molecules depends entirely on others. This is especially true with vitamins, which our body is not capable of producing and which are essential for generating other molecules that, in turn, are essential. This also happens when it comes to eliminating molecules that are essential to eliminate.

For example, B complex vitamins, like B6, B10, and B12, are essential to eliminate homocysteine, an oxidative molecule that is constantly produced by the metabolism of methionine [2].

The metabolic pathways in which these molecules transit and interrelate (move) are the subject of in-depth study through metabolomics and metabonomics [3]. Every day, science understands them a little more thanks to the generation of three-dimensional inter-systemic maps [4].

Movement at the Genetic and Chromosomal Level

Genetic and chromosomal movement not only occurs within a person, but the genetic material (the 'body' represented by the genes) is transported (moves) from one person to another at the moment of fertilisation, allowing the very foundations of life to be transformed: When a sperm fertilises an egg, two genetic stories of two different people travel generationally, making an intergenerational leap, a leap in movement in time, a leap in movement-time. We will return to this 'movement-time' issue in Chap. 9 of this book.

It is important to realise that failures in movement at any level will produce disorders that will influence other levels. These can be identified and managed by repair systems (e.g. one of the main functions of vitamin B12 is genetic repair) [5], or they can lead to diseases, some of them serious. Vitamin B12 deficiency, for example, causes hyperhomocysteinaemia, which is associated with osteoporosis and atherosclerosis [6, 7]. There are also times when failures in the movement of these systems produce conditions incompatible with extrauterine life, as occurs with some chromosomal problems.

To consolidate this new definition of 'movement' from the field of health a little, we will briefly return to kinematics and kinetics [8]:

Kinematics: the study of movement itself

Kinetics: the study of everything that can influence movement

These very brief definitions allow us to note that in life and health sciences we are interested in a complementary facet: the effects that movement has on the bodies that produce it (taking into account that body and movement are an indissoluble unit). Bodies, when moving/being in motion, bear consequences of said movement, which go far beyond changes in position in a spatial reference system.

The Intersection Between Health and Clinical Movement

We all know the definition of health: a state of complete biopsychosocial and functional well-being and not just the absence of disease [9]. Based on what has been stated regarding movement, we can venture a new definition and say that health is a 'state of perfect mobility'. This means that all systems, all components, and all bodies are in perfect motor balance. On the other hand, the disease can be understood as a result of altered, absent movements.

We will illustrate these concepts through a motor, physically motor example: the continuum of biological systems related to locomotion.

From the Molecule to the Interconnected System

Metabolic interactions between molecules allow the identification of metabolomic pathways, which, as they converge on their effectors, interrelate, and modulate each other. Calcium is the molecule of movement and, as such, the molecule of life: In fact, we can say that the **gold** standard of life is, in reality, a **calcium** standard. Just over 1.5% of our body is calcium, and this is considered to be a large and significant proportion: in a 65 kg person, it is equivalent to 1 kilo. Evolution established a 'central bank' of calcium in the bone skeleton, where 99% of the body's calcium is found as hydroxyapatite crystals. The remaining 1% is found in the blood, nervous tissue, and skeletal muscle [10].

In line with this, at the systemic level, we can identify pathways in which the included systems interrelate and modulate each other and are in turn capable of modulating the molecular world. If we look functionally at the distribution of calcium in our body, we see that practically 100% is distributed continuously, structurally, dynamically, and functionally in five systems: neurological, endocrine, musculoskeletal, bone, and haematological. We cannot understand any of the components of this continuum as 'independent' entities of one another. Rather, they are all interdependent.

We will call this continuum 'NEMOH': Neuro Endocrine Muscle Osseum Haematological [11].

Understanding its relationships allows us to understand how the system becomes ill, how to heal it, how to prevent its damage, and, once the damage is established, how to modulate its deterioration.

The Interconnected System and Its Molecules

Below, we give examples of deterioration conditions for each of the NEMOH components. These conditions are common in older people, but they are often underdiagnosed (or, even worse, underestimated).

Neurological

Vitamin B12 (cobalamin) [2] is water-soluble and has three main functions: genetic repair, elimination of homocysteine, and generation of the myelin sheath of peripheral neurons. This sheath allows electrochemical information to be transmitted in a saltatory manner, achieving speeds over 400 km/h. Thanks to this, postural reflexes exist. Without vitamin B12 and without myelin, bipedalism, one of the most characteristic evolutionary characteristics of human beings, could not have developed. This means, as we will explain below, that cobalamin deficiency is associated with falls, sarcopenia, and osteoporosis.

The degeneration of peripheral axons and soma due to the loss of myelin alters nerve conduction in speed and quality. The messages transmitted in the neuromuscular plate become equivocal and of inadequate intensity. This progressively alters muscle tone, from one myofibril to another, by altering its spatial and structural sequence and disordering its response capacity. This alters biomechanics by producing contractures and disorders of bone traction force vectors.

Endocrinological

Hyponatremia leads to the loss of the oncotic effect of sodium in the musculoskeletal capillary microenvironment, edematising the fibres, activating inflammatory pathways, and destroying the ecosystem or 'nest' of musculoskeletal stem cells (satellite cells). In this way, myofibres are lost, the myostatin pathway is activated and the necessary and usual repair processes are hindered. Thus, to the difficulty of maintaining oncotic pressures is added the loss of muscle, which in turn hinders venous return and generates oedema, producing a vicious circle [12].

This oncotic disaster is usually secondary to inadequate secretion of antidiuretic hormone (although it can also be due to the misuse of medications such as selective serotonin reuptake inhibitor antidepressants) and affects the entire NEMOH, producing orthostatism, falls, fear of falling, bruises, and fractures, reducing quality of life and functionality.

Muscles and Bone (Muscle-Osseum)

It might be thought that sarcopenia is the final stage of muscular deterioration, but it is, in turn, a cause of bone and musculoskeletal disorders. Indeed, sarcopenia produces a loss of muscle mass and strength, which alters the specificity of the specialisation in biomechanical patterns that muscle fibres have. This in turn produces disorders of the force vectors directed towards the bone tissue, generating osteopenia [13] and osteoporosis [14]. This translates into a disruption of the entire systems of older patients, being associated with an increase in falls, fractures, and mortality [15]. Similarly, osteopenia and osteoporosis lead to greater sarcopenia, although the pathways are not fully defined [16].

Haematological

Iron is a key element in transporting oxygen and synthesising collagen, haemoglobin, myoglobin, myelin, neurotransmitters, and components of the mitochondrial electron transport chain. Older people frequently suffer from iron deficiency. Its main causes are low intake of foods rich in iron, disorders in absorption and transport, and chronic losses [17]. Iron deficiency activates various inflammatory pathways, causing serious disorders such as anaemia, sarcopenia, muscle atrophy, osteoporosis, and cognitive and cardiovascular disorders [18–20]. Iron deficiency is an independent risk factor for fatigue and poor functional recovery in older people [21]. In this way, and due to its high prevalence in older people, iron deficiency is positioned as one of the main risk factors for the haematological bone-muscle neuroendocrine continuum in older people.

Frailty and Continuous Motion Concept

All these concepts are in line and closely related with the concept of 'frailty', understood as a multisystemic impairment with minor and major alterations, in addition to organ diseases, that erode the vital capacity or system functional reserve leading to failure of the machinery in generating the energy to sustain appropriate micro-movements and organ-system interaction and in generating the failure to thrive [22].

Movement, as we are presenting, is a major key to understanding and clinically applying concepts such as frailty. Movement is constantly present throughout the human bioeconomy, at all levels of the body and mind, and in the social and functional dimension, even in the spiritual one.

To understand how movement 'flows', it is good to consider continuums like the NEMOH [11]. NEMOH has evolved and has been perfected to facilitate our movements. Muscle chains (circuits of muscles and fascia, in continuity of direction and planes, that work together and in a coordinated manner to distribute and propagate forces through the human body to maintain posture and adapt movement) are another type of 'continuum' [23].

For each continuum, there are movements that protect health and allow optimising the aging process, generating healthy aging. Likewise, there are deleterious movements, which negatively affect the 'biological economy'/the health economy and produce pathological aging [24]. On the other hand, insufficient muscle activity, in itself a form of pathological movement, alters muscle metabolism and generates a true vicious circle, especially harmful in older people [25].

We can say that there is an intrinsic difficulty in maintaining the correction of all the characteristics (intention, coordination, rhythm, direction, speed, etc.) of all the movements present in a body, or in a group of bodies (e.g., a human society). Then, just one 'little' problem in 'just' one characteristic will affect all the 'moving system' and, if not repaired with 'repairing movements', will transform the life 'dance' into uncoordinated movements, transforming 'pleasant' time in 'suffering' time: illness. However, the disease can also appear because of lack of mobility, as occurs massively in sedentary society.

On the other hand, healthy lifestyles, exercise, and physiotherapy can be considered 'correct' movements. They have great positive impacts on the health of the entire bioeconomy, particularly when they are part of healthy aging strategies and are directed with prophylactic and/or therapeutic intent on people or the population. Indeed, their impact is not merely mechanical and 'macro', but they are capable of, for example, influencing the mitochondrial machinery to make it more effective and efficient, generating fewer oxygen free radicals. Thus, they have a virtuous effect on inflammatory cascades and other harmful forms of pathological movement. Exercise can upregulate muscle mitochondrial homeostasis and enhance antioxidant capacity, representing an effective way to prevent muscle—and NEMOH—deterioration [26].

References

1. de la Torre Zermeño FJ. El mundo de la Física 1. Tema 6, el Movimiento como cambio de lugar en función del tiempo. México City: Editorial Progreso; 2003. p. 74.
2. López LJ, Dinamarca-Montecinos JL, Mejía-Rojas K, Cuadros ACB, Bárcena JBA, Palacios-Sánchez L, Fernandez-Fairen M. Vitamins B1, B6, and B12 and peripheral neuropathies: international expert consensus. Revista de la Facultad de Medicina Humana. 2024;24(1):12. https://doi.org/10.25176/RFMH.v24i1.6413. https://inicib.urp.edu.pe/rfmh/vol24/iss1/12.
3. Nicholson JK, Holmes E, Lindon JC. Chapter 1—Metabonomics and metabolomics techniques and their applications in mammalian systems. In: Lindon JC, Nicholson JK, Holmes E, editors. The handbook of meta-

bonomics and metabolomics. Elsevier Science B.V.; 2007. p. 1–33. https://doi.org/10.1016/B978-044452841-4/50002-3.
4. Akhbari P, Karamchandani U, Jaggard MKJ, Graça G, Bhattacharya R, Lindon JC, Williams HRT, Gupte CM. Can joint fluid metabolic profiling (or "metabonomics") reveal biomarkers for osteoarthritis and inflammatory joint disease? A systematic review. Bone Jt Res. 2020;9(3):108–19. https://doi.org/10.1302/2046-3758.93.BJR-2019-0167.R1.
5. Praveen G, Sivaprasad M, Reddy GB. Telomere length and vitamin B12. Vitam Horm. 2022;119:299–324. https://doi.org/10.1016/bs.vh.2022.01.014.
6. Zaric BL, Obradovic M, Bajic V, Haidara MA, Jovanovic M, Isenovic ER. Homocysteine and hyperhomocysteinaemia. Curr Med Chem. 2019;26(16):2948–61. https://doi.org/10.2174/092986732566618031310 5949.
7. Tinelli C, Di Pino A, Ficulle E, Marcelli S, Feligioni M. Hyperhomocysteinemia as a risk factor and potential nutraceutical target for certain pathologies. Front Nutr. 2019;6(6):49. https://doi.org/10.3389/fnut.2019.00049.
8. Borel, M., Vénizélos, G. (2016). Chapters 2 and 3: Movement equations 1: location, kinematics and kinetics. Wiley
9. Schramme T. Health as complete well-being: the WHO definition and beyond. Public Health Ethics. 2023;16(3):210–8. https://doi.org/10.1093/phe/phad017.
10. Ross AC, Taylor CL, Yaktine AL, et al., editors. Institute of Medicine (US) Committee to review dietary reference intakes for vitamin D and calcium. Dietary reference intakes for calcium and vitamin D. Washington (DC): National Academies Press (US); 2011. https://doi.org/10.17226/13050. https://www.ncbi.nlm.nih.gov/books/NBK56070/.
11. Luis D-MJ. Chapter 33—Enfermedades musculoesqueléticas. In: d'Hyver C, Robledo LMG, Gil CHZ, editors. Geriatría. México City: Editorial El Manual Moderno; 2024.
12. Fujisawa C, Umegaki H, Sugimoto T, Samizo S, Huang CH, Fujisawa H, et al. Mild hyponatremia is associated with low skeletal muscle mass, physical function impairment, and depressive mood in the elderly. BMC Geriatr. 2021;21(1):15. https://doi.org/10.1186/s12877-020-01955-4.
13. Teng Z, Zhu Y, Yu X, Liu J, Long Q, Zeng Y, Lu S. An analysis and systematic review of sarcopenia increasing osteopenia risk. PLoS One. 2021;16(4):e0250437. https://doi.org/10.1371/journal.pone.0250437.
14. Lee DY, Shin S. Association of sarcopenia with osteopenia and osteoporosis in community-dwelling older Korean adults: a cross-sectional study. J Clin Med. 2021;11(1):129. https://doi.org/10.3390/jcm11010129.
15. Salech F, Marquez C, Lera L, Angel B, Saguez R, Albala C. Osteosarcopenia predicts falls, fractures, and mortality in Chilean community-dwelling older adults. J Am Med Dir Assoc. 2021;22:853–8. https://doi.org/10.1016/j.jamda.2020.07.032.

16. Edwards M, Dennison E, Sayer AA, Fielding R, Cooper C. Osteoporosis and sarcopenia in older age. Bone. 2015;80:126–30. https://doi.org/10.1016/j.bone.2015.04.016.
17. Zeidan RS, Han SM, Leeuwenburgh C, Xiao R. Iron homeostasis and organismal aging. Ageing Res Rev. 2021;72:101510. https://doi.org/10.1016/j.arr.2021.101510.
18. Krabbe KS, Pedersen M, Bruunsgaard H. Inflammatory mediators in the elderly. Exp Gerontol. 2004;39:687–99. https://doi.org/10.1016/j.exger.2004.01.009.
19. DeRuisseau KC, Park Y-M, DeRuisseau LR, Cowley PM, Fazen CH, Doyle RP. Aging-related changes in the iron status of skeletal muscle. Exp Gerontol. 2013;48:1294–302. https://doi.org/10.1016/j.exger.2013.08.011.
20. Kim TH, Hwang H-J, Kim S-H. Relationship between serum ferritin levels and sarcopenia in Korean females aged 60 years and older using the fourth Korea National Health and Nutrition Examination Survey (KNHANES IV-2, 3), 2008–2009. PLoS One. 2014;9:e90105. https://doi.org/10.1371/journal.pone.0090105.
21. Neidlein S, Wirth R, Pourhassan M. Iron deficiency, fatigue and muscle strength and function in older hospitalized patients. Eur J Clin Nutr. 2021;75(3):456–63. https://doi.org/10.1038/s41430-020-00742-z.
22. Chen X, Mao G, Leng SX. Frailty syndrome: an overview. Clin Interv Aging. 2014;9:433–41. https://doi.org/10.2147/CIA.S45300.
23. Busquet L. CADENAS MUSCULARES, LAS (Tomo I). Tronco y columna cervical. Barcelona: Paidotribo; 2007.
24. Dinamarca-Montecinos JL, Rubio-Herrera R, Bonta-Arias C, de la Dismovilidad T. Movimiento, tiempo y envejecimiento. En búsqueda de las bases de una única teoría del envejecimiento. Beca Mapfre de Investigación; 2007. https://documentacion.fundacionmapfre.org/documentacion/publico/es/bib/131894.do?queryId=49308.
25. Rezuş E, Burlui A, Cardoneanu A, Rezuş C, Codreanu C, Pârvu M, Rusu Zota G, Tamba BI. Inactivity and skeletal muscle metabolism: a vicious cycle in old age. Int J Mol Sci. 2020;21:592. https://doi.org/10.3390/ijms21020592.
26. Li J, Wang Z, Li C, Song Y, Wang Y, Bo H, Zhang Y. Impact of exercise and aging on mitochondrial homeostasis in skeletal muscle: roles of ROS and epigenetics. Cells. 2022;11(13):2086. https://doi.org/10.3390/cells11132086.

2 The Great Geriatric Syndromes and the Immobility Syndrome

The History, Concept, and Characteristics of Geriatric Syndromes

The aging process has been part of human concern since ancient times. Human beings have recognised both its negative effects—such as the loss of autonomy and difficulty in getting around—and its positive effects, such as experience and wisdom. Other elements associated with aging, such as longevity and death, have also been the subject of profound discussions over time.

In the field of health and healthcare, gerontology emerged as an area of study at the end of the nineteenth century, while geriatrics emerged as a conceptual proposal in 1906 and clinical in the mid-1940s. The main tools proposed then to facilitate geriatric practice were interdisciplinarity, comprehensive care, definition of daily living activities, protection of functional independence, creation of clinical units specialised services, and early mobilisation of patients admitted to hospitals [1].

At the end of the 1960s, the concept of 'Giants of Geriatrics' and the mnemonic of the '4i' were proposed: immobility, instability, cognitive problems, and incontinence [2].

J. L. Dinamarca-Montecinos, *Dysmobility in Geriatrics*, https://doi.org/10.1007/978-3-031-72716-0_2

A Definition of Geriatric Syndrome

From Lionel Cosin's hip fractures during the Second World War [3], the defunctionalisation of patients proposed by Marjory Warren in 1940 [4], the orthogeriatrics of Michael Devas and Robert Irvine in the 1960s [5], and the so-called '4i's' by Bernard Isaacs in the early 1970s [2], the number and complexity of syndromes considered geriatric has been increasing more and more. Today, not only syndromes of biological or mental origin are proposed but also social (e.g. abuse, abandonment, empty nest) [6] and spiritual syndromes (e.g. fear of death, crisis of faith) [7, 8].

Although the concept of 'geriatric syndrome' is part of the core of geriatrics, it has not been fully defined, and its understanding is quite heterogeneous [9]. Some works have used specific syndromes to generate models which make it easier to identify when a syndrome really is a geriatric syndrome [10].

In general, to be considered 'geriatric', in addition to being a set of signs and symptoms of diverse aetiology, a syndrome must meet some essential characteristics. A geriatric syndrome must be:

- Highly prevalent in geriatric ages[1] (usually over 60 years) (and/or have a minimal or much lower representation in younger ages).
- Multifactorial.
- Necessarily managed at various levels of care, to be sustainable. This involves preventive, acute, rehabilitation, and follow-up aspects, not only in the clinical field but also in the political-organisational field.
- A final characteristic of geriatric syndromes is linked to the relationship that the syndromes maintain with geriatrics. Typically, individuals who present with a 'geriatric syndrome'

[1] **Note**: Age is seen as an epidemiological-associated criterion, ***never*** an etiological one. That is, age is a cut-off point to relate geriatric syndromes to the older population and differentiate their frequency with respect to the younger population, but it is not age that defines their appearance.

and are managed with a geriatrics approach have evidence of better results (particularly in functionality and quality of life) than those who are managed with 'usual' or 'traditional' management.

This forces us to briefly summarise the characteristics of geriatrics management. We will do it according to four commonly used 'geriatric' historic concepts:

- Integrality: According to the biopsychosocial, spiritual, and functional paradigm.
- Interdisciplinarity: Several disciplines working together.
- Various levels: Cover all levels of care, not only outpatient and hospital but also home, community, and the interfaces between them, which are called 'liaison'.
- Staging: A description of the natural history of diseases, based on the definition of key stages. These stages are turning points when it is necessary to intervene to reverse, slow, or stop the progression of a disease. This is an important element of a proactive approach and management in geriatrics [11].

Along with this, we have defined four characteristics to better characterise when a syndrome is geriatric, based on its natural history [12]:

1. *Self-perpetuation*: Each consequence of a geriatric syndrome negatively influences others and itself. This can generate vicious circles that make recovery difficult, rather than facilitating the progression of the disease.
2. *Descending progression*: Or 'downward sloping' effect. The natural history of geriatric syndromes inevitably evolves towards loss of functionality, dependency, and death if interventions are not carried out in time. Outcomes become progressively worse. Older people don't 'get better on their own', and the outcomes of geriatric syndromes don't improve on their own.

3. *Contagiousness*: Geriatric syndromes have the capacity to progressively compromise social levels, from the intimacy of the family to the integrity of health systems.
4. *Expansiveness*: Or 'cluster bomb' effect. One geriatric syndrome will lead to the appearance of other geriatric syndromes. Geriatric syndromes are associated with each other and attack various systems that apparently have nothing to do with each other.

Immobility Syndrome

Definitions of Immobility Syndrome

As we have seen, immobility syndrome has long been considered one of the so-called 'giants of geriatrics', and one of the classic 'i's' of geriatrics corresponds to it.

Some classic definitions of immobility syndrome, immobility or immobilisation, consist of:

> *'Decrease in the ability to perform activities of daily living due to deterioration of motor functions. It is characterized by reduced tolerance to physical capacity, progressive muscle weakness and, in severe cases, loss of automatisms and postural reflexes necessary for ambulation'.* [13]

> *'Restriction, generally involuntary, in the transfer and/or displacement capacity of a person due to physical, functional, or psychosocial problems'.* [14]

Strengths and Weaknesses of the Definition of Immobility Syndrome

These definitions have some strengths and weaknesses, which we review below:

Strengths

They allow us to recognise the existence of a syndrome that is characterised by motor problems.

They recognise not just motor aetiology but also psychosocial ones.

They allow large groups of patients affected by these conditions to be diagnosed.

Weaknesses

'Immobility', that is, the absolute absence of movement, does not exist.

There tends to be confusion between 'mobility' and 'functionality'.

Common definitions of immobility do not consider the condition of the motor continuum, so they do not allow:

(a) Early motor alterations to be recognised
(b) The stages of motor disorders to be associated with other diseases
(c) Grouping according to evolution and prognosis
(d) Comparing groups of patients or treatment groups
(e) Standardised correlation with quality of life

Table 2.1 summarises some points regarding the scope and limitations of the classic definitions of immobility syndrome.

Table 2.1 Scope and limitations of the classic definitions of immobility syndrome

Area	Classic definitions of immobility syndrome	
	Allows	Does not allow
Clinics	Identify patients in severe stages Identify large, homogeneous groups of patients Generate general guidelines regarding management Establish short-term prognosis in individual patients in the acute phase, especially terminal	Identify patients in the early stages Identify subgroups of patients according to aetiology, evolution, and prognosis Compare and standardise management based on patient series Standardise and limit prognoses, between short, medium, and long terms, based on patient series
Research	Describe large groups of subjects with the syndrome Monocentric statistical comparisons	Describe, define, and establish specific groups Multicentre statistical comparison in relation to the evolution of patient series

References

1. Howell TH. Origins of British geriatrics. Proc R Soc Med. 1976;69(6):445–9. PMID: 785477; PMCID: PMC1864279.
2. Felstein I. A giant of geriatric medicine—Professor Bernard Isaacs (1924–1995) Post 1. https://www.bgs.org.uk/a-giant-of-geriatric-medicine-professor-bernard-isaacs-1924-1995-post-1.
3. Barton A, Mulley G. History of the development of geriatric medicine in the UK. Postgrad Med J. 2003;79(930):229–34; quiz 233–4. https://doi.org/10.1136/pmj.79.930.229.
4. St John PD, Hogan DB. The relevance of Marjory Warren's writings today. Gerontologist. 2014;54(1):21–9. https://doi.org/10.1093/geront/gnt053.
5. Devas MB. Geriatric orthopaedics. Br Med J. 1974;1(5900):190–2.
6. Wang G, Hu M, Xiao SY, Zhou L. Loneliness and depression among rural empty-nest elderly adults in Liuyang, China: a cross-sectional study. BMJ Open. 2017;7(10):e016091. https://doi.org/10.1136/bmjopen-2017-016091.
7. Coelho-Júnior HJ, Calvani R, Panza F, Allegri RF, Picca A, Marzetti E, Alves VP. Religiosity/spirituality and mental health in older adults: a systematic review and meta-analysis of observational studies. Front Med (Lausanne). 2022;9:877213. https://doi.org/10.3389/fmed.2022.877213.
8. Upenieks L. Uncertainty in faith, fear of death? Transitions in religious doubt and death anxiety in later life. Omega (Westport). 2023;87(3):814–37. https://doi.org/10.1177/00302228211029475.
9. Olde Rikkert MG, Rigaud AS, van Hoeyweghen RJ, de Graaf J. Geriatric syndromes: medical misnomer or progress in geriatrics? Neth J Med. 2003;61(3):83–7.
10. Inouye SK, Studenski S, Tinetti ME, Kuchel GA. Geriatric syndromes: clinical, research, and policy implications of a core geriatric concept. J Am Geriatr Soc. 2007;55(5):780–91. https://doi.org/10.1111/j.1532-5415.2007.01156.x.
11. Sennour Y, Counsell SR, Jones J, Weiner M. Development and implementation of a proactive geriatrics consultation model in collaboration with hospitalists. J Am Geriatr Soc. 2009;57(11):2139–45. https://doi.org/10.1111/j.1532-5415.2009.02496.x.
12. Dinamarca-Montecinos JL. Dysmobility in geriatrics. A decade defining a clinical concept. Bol Hosp Vina del Mar, 2012 68(2):15–19
13. Jimenez Rojas C, Carrillo Manrique B. Manual de Geriatría Salgado Alba. 3rd ed. Barcelona: Editorial Masson; 2002.
14. González Montalvo JI, Alarcón Alarcón T. Great geriatric syndromes, concept and prevention of the most important ones. Medicine. 2003;8(108):5778–85.

3 Reconceptualisation of Immobility: Dysmobility

Reconceptualising: From Immobility to Dysmobility

We have seen the strengths and weaknesses of the classic definitions of immobility syndrome, and we have also seen that there is little difference between them. Based on this, we can complement these definitions with etiological, diagnostic, evolutionary, therapeutic, and prognostic elements:

(a) **Etiological**: It is necessary to consider all possible origins, not only biological alterations but also mental, social, and spiritual ones. The latter, is an under-explored area by medicine, which may acquire special relevance in older people.
(b) **Diagnostics**: Measure motor capacity and not just independence. Mobility is not limited to the exclusive scope of activities of daily living (ADLs). ADLs are an important standard for measuring quality of life, but daily life is more than its activities, whether they are basic, instrumental, advanced, recreational, productive, or whatever the classification used.
(c) **Evolutionary**: It is necessary to use staging to define ranges and stages. This will allow intervention to (1) prevent progression to deeper stages, (2) study the prognosis and define the best management according to each stage; (3) include subjects with transient etiology (apparently inconsequential), and (4) include subjects who, without having a decrease in

J. L. Dinamarca-Montecinos, *Dysmobility in Geriatrics*,
https://doi.org/10.1007/978-3-031-72716-0_3

their motor capabilities, can perform their movements but with varying degrees of discomfort.

(d) **Therapeutics**: Concept of locomotion and transfer. The word 'locomotion' comes from the Latin *locus* (place) and *motio* (movement) and refers to the possibility of changing 'place' intentionally. The mere use of the term 'movement' does not necessarily consider the meaning and the 'why' the motor *intention*.

People move not only because they want to but because it is inherent to the nature of all things: whether we like it or not, we are 'in motion', because we unconsciously move parts of our organism or because many parts of it move reflexively or not voluntary.

Our volitional capacity leads us to decide to perform or not perform certain movements. Many of the movements of living beings are the expression of motor intentions, the result of a cognitive-motor process. Also, one of the ways of expressing these intentions is to change places—whether physically, cognitively, socially, or spiritually.

This expands the diagnostic and management possibilities, since the 'transfer' is usually the really important part of the 'why' of motor intention: What do we gain by being able to 'move' without being able to 'transfer'? Or, even better, what do we gain by being able to 'move' without achieving what we want to?

(e) **Prognostic**: Progression concept. The concept of progression is characteristic of geriatric syndromes, based on the natural history of the pathology over the passage of time. This would allow an outcome or ending result (an 'immobilized' patient) to be transformed into a process (a patient suffering one or other stage of Dysmobility), which can be evaluated at initial stages, allowing early intervention to prevent the geriatric syndrome from progressing.

Definition of Dysmobility

Given the literature and debate presented in previous chapters, we can conclude that we need to redefine the concept of immobility syndrome.

Dysmobility

The annoyance, difficulty and/or impossibility of mobilizing part of the body and/or of relocating/transferring oneself from one place to another secondary to various pathological situations from any origin (biological, psychological, social, spiritual, functional, etc.) that affects the quality of life and/or that have risk of progression.

The next section will reconceptualise Immobility as 'Dysmobility', which we will define as:

Annoying mobility: That which allows the desired to be achieved with discomfort, but without altering the normal course of movement or without the need to resort to neighboring motor functional units or global compensation [1]

Difficult mobility: That which allows one to achieve what is desired but which alters the normal physical course of movement

Both (annoyance and difficulty) are independent of the causes, which can be very varied. For example, pain, absence of a limb, vertigo, dyspnea, etc.

This definition complements the classic ones in the following points:

(a) **Etiological**: It does not exclude any possible origin. Any element can disrupt mobility, causing Dysmobility. When we identify Dysmobility, we must intervene. It does not matter if it is transitory or 'very initial'.
(b) **Diagnostics**: The diagnostic process is simplified, since we can focus on a standardised diagnostic method, as we will see later.

(c) **Evolutionary**: Evolutionary aspects of the definition include three aspects: (1) Optimises diagnostic accuracy by including three ranges (annoyance, difficulty, and impossibility), instead of just 'decline'. This allows patients with transient illnesses to be included. (2) By including quality of life, it allows us to visualize the natural history of the syndrome and not just its final stages. (3) This, in turn, will allow us to relate these stages to specific etiologies and complications.
(d) **Therapeutics**: Clearly defined etiologies and complications associated with evolutionary stages allow the standardization of therapeutic, preventive, and screening processes.
(e) **Prognostic**: By allowing comparison between different therapeutic methods for the same stage and etiology, the corresponding functional and motor prognosis can be defined with much greater certainty.

Keynote

Dysmobility and other terms: prostration, movement dysfunction, and dysfunctional movements

Prostration: This word comes from the Latin '*postrare*', which literally means '*to kneel*'. It refers imprecisely to a serious loss of motor ability. This can be involuntary and catastrophic (leads the person to dependency) or voluntary and marital (associated with religious practices or requests for clemency). However, its use does not have a clear origin in clinical practice.

It is possible that in theocentric antiquity, the occurrence of serious traumatic accidents or the birth of people with serious illnesses may have been seen as a kind of divine punishment, which led the person who suffered them to be in a position to ask for forgiveness, that is, say 'prostrate', 'kneeling', due to a shortening of the flexor muscles of the lower extremities.

This concept would have been progressively adopted, associated with terminal illness conditions, currently becoming directly associated with older people.

There are some drawbacks when using non-technical or descriptive terms, with imprecise definitions, and that imply emotional charges, in health, as is the case of 'prostration'.

- The first is that they do not specify a stage exactly: How many types of 'prostration' are there? What is the prognosis for each type of 'prostration'? What message exactly does the clinician want to deliver when referring to a patient being 'prostrate'?
- The second is that it can carry a significant pejorative burden and generate a negative impact on the caregivers, the patient, and even the health team: It is very different to say that a patient is in stage 5-A of recent acute Dysmobility secondary to a right ischemic stroke than to say that the patient 'was left prostrate'. In the first case, precise technical information is provided, linking causes with processes, stages, treatments, and prognoses. In the second, there is only talk in a non-technical way of a catastrophic state.
- The third is that a clinician cannot obtain any objective information about a diagnosis of 'prostration'. Each clinician will understand what seems to him according to the case, according to his experience, or according to other circumstances. This generates heterogeneity of interpretations about the diagnosis, which can affect the general management of the patient.

After reading the previous chapters, we can establish that the term 'prostration' does not constitute a medical diagnosis or a health diagnosis. Perhaps it could be used for political or marital purposes but not in a technical field that seeks to establish processes that link certain etiologies with certain forms of evolution, treatment, and prognosis. This is why we suggest avoiding the use of the term 'prostration' in health. Also, in geriatrics, in particular, it should be replaced by a correct diagnosis of Dysmobility syndrome.

Movement dysfunction: This expression does not relate to *motor capacity* (mobility) but refers to movement as a separate entity, independent of the bodies that move. However, we have seen that movement does not exist except in relation to the 'bodies that move'. So, it is not entirely correct to speak of movement dysfunction but rather of *mobility* dysfunctions, that is, of different forms of Dysmobility.

Dysfunctional movements: On the other hand, 'dysfunctional movements' can be considered part of certain types of Dysmobility, as they could consist of voluntary movements that fail to generate the desired result (i.e. osteoarthritis) or involuntary movements that are signs of several conditions with more or less specific etiologies (i.e. Parkinson's disease).

Reference

1. Busquets L. Las cadenas musculares, tomo II. Chapter 2: El Movimiento, Unidades Funcionales. 6th ed. Barcelona: Editorial Paidotribo; 2005. p. 44–6.

Diagnosis of Dysmobility: The Triaxial Diagnosis Method

4

The Triaxial Diagnosis Method

Like any geriatric syndrome, Dysmobility benefits from a diagnosis that includes cross-sectional and longitudinal views on the time axis. In this way, the diagnosis of Dysmobility must be made in a triaxial manner, including the speed of installation, the time of evolution, and its staging.

Axis 1. Speed of Installation

Dysmobility can establish abruptly, in a fast and acute manner, or slowly, being even not evident for a long time.

We will understand 'acute' and 'fast' in its meaning related to something that emerges in a very short time, which is why it becomes evident 'abruptly', in a cross-section of time. For the opposite, 'slow', we will understand in the sense that it takes a long time to become evident, which can be noticed with a longitudinal look at the time. Then, note that 'slow' (something that evolves at a low speed) does not mean 'chronic' (something which lasts a lifetime).

Therefore, we have two types of Dysmobility: Acute (fast, abrupt) Dysmobility, and Slow Dysmobility. The characteristics of both types of Dysmobility are presented in Table 4.1.

J. L. Dinamarca-Montecinos, *Dysmobility in Geriatrics*,
https://doi.org/10.1007/978-3-031-72716-0_4

Table 4.1 Characteristics of slow and acute Dysmobility

Dysmobility	Slow	Acute (fast, abrupt)
Speed and form of presentation	**Slow and hypocritical, sometimes subclinical**	**Acute, usually spectacular, always evident**
Aetiology	Multiple associated underlying chronic diseases	Acute homeostatic failure
Clinical presentation	Signs and symptoms with high variability over time and non-specific evolution in the long term	Quite specific and obvious. Characteristic evolution in a short time
Diagnostic history	The patient and family/caregivers have different opinions about the origin of their symptoms The patient 'lives' with the symptoms for a long time before a diagnosis is made	The patient and family/caregivers suspect the same diagnosis with a high level of certainty In a very short time, at least a syndromic diagnosis is established
Diagnostic level of care	Generally ambulatory or domiciliary	High percentage in emergency units
Therapeutic response	Good response to medical-pharmacological management and healthy lifestyles	Variable response to acute treatment
Prognostic	It can be complicated by Acute (fast, abrupt) Dysmobility Low secondary mortality	High probability of sequelae, complications, and relapses High secondary morbidity and mortality

Based on Dinamarca-Montecinos JL. Dysmobility in Geriatrics. A decade defining a clinical concept. Bol Hosp Vina del Mar, 2012 68(2):15–19 [1]

Axis 2. Evolution Time

Dysmobility can be old or recent, since the onset of symptoms. We have proposed as the limit of this division, 1 year from the onset of symptoms: At 1 year, the Dysmobility becomes old. One year is a suitable cut-off point to demarcate recent and old because at 1 year post onset of Dysmobility, it becomes more difficult to improve, and further complications are more likely. Thus, after 1 year, the prognosis and therapeutic approach vary greatly. For more information about regression and progression of Dysmobility, see Chap. 5.

Both forms of presentation of Dysmobility can be aetiologically related, although this is not always the case. It is more common for slow Dysmobility to be complicated by acute Dysmobility. For example, osteoarthritis and obstructive lung disease—typical examples of conditions that generate slowly evolving Dysmobility—can be complicated by falls, fractures, and respiratory infections, all examples of Acute Dysmobility. This gives rise to Mixed Dysmobility.

A graphic representation of Slow and Acute Dysmobility can be seen in Graphics 4.1 and 4.2.

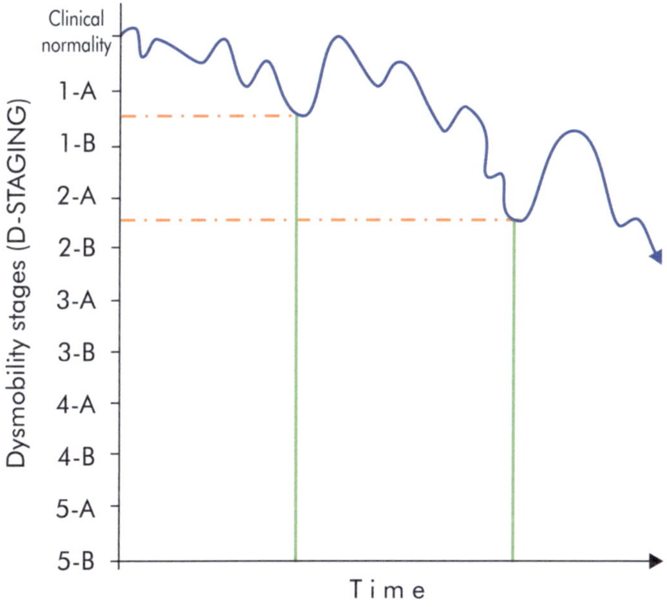

Graphic 4.1 Natural evolution of slow Dysmobility and response after starting motor rehabilitation (*). *Based on Dinamarca-Montecinos JL. Dysmobility in Geriatrics. A decade defining a clinical concept. Bol Hosp Vina del Mar, 2012 68(2):15–19 [1]

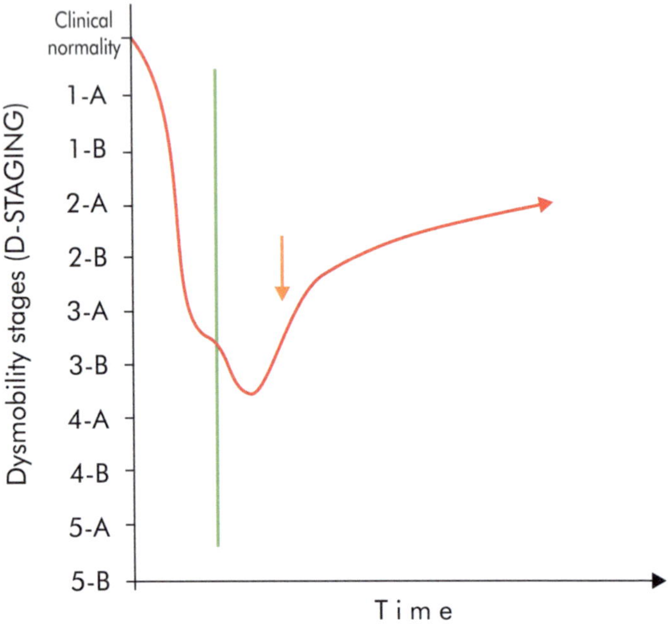

Graphic 4.2 Natural evolution of acute Dysmobility and response after starting in-hospital rehabilitation (*). *Based on Dinamarca Montecinos JL. De la Inmovilidad a la Dismovilidad en Geriatría. Ediciones de la Sociedad Chilena de Psicogeriatría, Santiago, Chile, 2004 [2]

The blue line shows a slow loss of locomotor capacity, with remissions and exacerbations that are difficult to perceive but constantly progress towards increasingly deeper stages of Dysmobility. Successive symptomatic measures on non-specific diagnoses are usually implemented at times of major motor loss (orange lines), such as the passage from stage 1-A to 1-B (use of walking stick, occurrence of falls) or from 2-A to 2-B (difficulty getting up from the chair). In the short term, they have beneficial effects, but they are generally abandoned, and between the implementation of one and the other, the consolidation of locomotor deterioration is noticeable (green lines).

The red line shows a rapid loss of motor ability. Short time elapses between the acute event and the moment of diagnosis (green line). There may be functional recovery if interdisciplinary rehabilitation treatment is instituted in a short time.

Axis 3. Staging

Dysmobility staging is carried out through D-STAGING, a dynamic system (continuum). D-STAGING is knowing as ETADI in Spanish.

D-STAGING consists of five stages with two substages each, giving a total of ten substages.

The description of the process can be seen in D-STAGING, in Table 4.2:

Table 4.2 D-STAGING

		Stages				
		1	2	3	4	5
		The patient				
				Remains in bed most of the day		
		Stands most of the day	Remain sitting most of the day	Moves in bed and out of bed	Moves in bed	Does not move
Substages	A	Walks without help	Sits and stands up alone	The patient gets out of bed, alone or with help	Moves upper and lower extremities and/or can make turns	Expresses himself/herself, makes herself/himself understood
	B	Walks with help (technical aids or help from third parties. Includes walking while leaning on furniture or walls)	Needs help sitting and/or getting up	Sits on the edge of the bed, alone or with help	Moves upper or lower extremities Needs help making turns	Does not express himself, he does not make himself understood

Based on Dinamarca-Montecinos JL. Dysmobility in Geriatrics. A decade defining a clinical concept. Bol Hosp Vina del Mar, 2012 68(2):15–19 [1]; Dinamarca Montecinos JL. De la Inmovilidad a la Dismovilidad en Geriatría. Ediciones de la Sociedad Chilena de Psicogeriatría, Santiago, Chile, 2004 [2]

Types of Dysmobility

There are three types of Dysmobility:

- RAD (Recent Acute Dysmobility)
- OAD (Old Acute Dysmobility)
- OSD (Old Slow Dysmobility)

The diagnosis of Mixed Dysmobility (slow and acute) can be considered but referring to both types separately.

Complementary Notes

It is interesting to consider the prognosis of Dysmobility: permanent or temporary. A sprained ankle, for example, with good rehabilitation will have *restitutio ad integrum*, which will generate acute, recent, and transitory Dysmobility.

The 'depth' of Dysmobility increases as the stages increase. In this way, we can refer to stage 5 as 'deep' Dysmobility, although there is no such thing as 'superficial' Dysmobility.

From a clinical point of view, it is convenient to consider Recent Slow Dysmobility as a subtype of Old Slow Dysmobility. This is because at the time of clinical diagnosis, it will already have a long evolution time.

References

1. Dinamarca-Montecinos JL. Dysmobility in geriatrics. A decade defining a clinical concept. Bol Hosp Vina del Mar, 2012 68(2):15–19
2. Dinamarca Montecinos JL. De la Inmovilidad a la Dismovilidad en Geriatría. Santiago: Ediciones de la Sociedad Chilena de Psicogeriatría; 2004.

Concepts of D-STAGING and Stability

5

The Dysmobility Continuum

The ten substages of D-STAGING can be conceptually summarised in three basic categories of mobility in the natural history of Dysmobility: pedalism (standing), sedentarism (sitting), and being bed-bound.

This dysmobilising continuum can be seen in Fig. 5.1:

The arrow represents the temporal axis, in which N = normality and the different substages of Dysmobility are linked together, forming a *dysmobilising process*. Note that the sitting stages (2-A and 2-B) form an intermediate stage between life in a standing position and lying in bed.

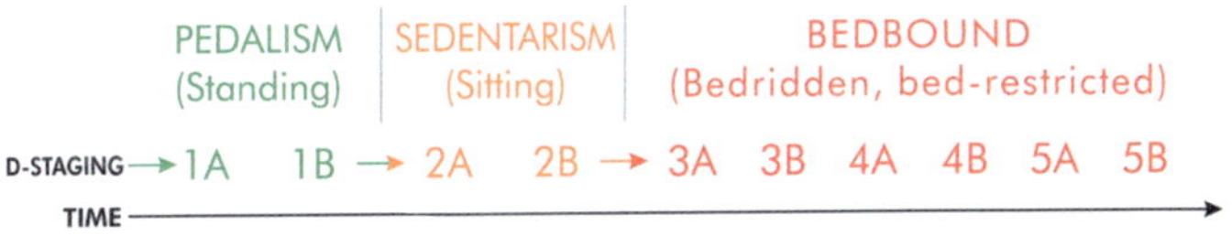

Fig. 5.1 Dysmobility continuum in older people (*). Based on Dinamarca-Montecinos JL. Dysmobility in Geriatrics. A decade defining a clinical concept. Bol Hosp Vina del Mar, 2012;68(2):15–19 [1]

J. L. Dinamarca-Montecinos, *Dysmobility in Geriatrics*,
https://doi.org/10.1007/978-3-031-72716-0_5

By ordering these moments of the evolution of Dysmobility with the stages, we obtain:

- Stage 1: Patient in category 1, pedalism (with standing life)
- Stage 2: Patient in category 2, sedentarism
- Stages3, 4, and 5: Patient who is bed-bound

This description of the natural history of Dysmobility allows two moments of dramatic clinical difference to be made evident, between stages 1 and 2 and between stages 2 and 3. This leaves the sitting stage as a hinge between the standing stages and lying-in-bed ones.

On the other hand, substage B are more serious than substage A since they are the prelude to the next stage. Substage A describes better mobility and greater motor independence, while substage B describes worse mobility and greater motor dependence.

In this way, substage A tends to be a substage of stabilisation and better prognosis, and substage B tends to be transitional, with a more complex prognosis.

In substage A, the therapeutic objective will be to return to the previous stage. For example, if the patient is in bed stage 4-A, return to sitting stage 2-B.

In substage B, the main objectives will be to achieve stabilisation and prevent progression to the next stage.

Prognosis: Time of Management and Concept of Stability

By integrating time into the prognosis of dysmobilised patients, we seek to emphasise that Dysmobility, being a geriatric syndrome, has a natural history of a continuum in permanent progression: The deterioration curve can only improve or stabilise due to the intervention of health and social care professionals.

Stability includes 3 possible scenarios, which are mutually exclusive: progression of Dysmobility towards deeper stages, whereas stabilisation and regression can move the Dysmobility towards earlier stages.

Patients in Substage A

For patients in substage A, four phases are considered:

- **In progression**: During the first 6 months after diagnosis, Dysmobility should be considered in progression towards the next substages.

  Based on the characteristics of geriatric syndromes, it is important to clarify that this does not mean that during this 6-month period, Dysmobility will *necessarily progress until taking the patient to a new substage*. Rather, if adequate management is not implemented, the deterioration curve will continue to decline, progressively increasing the risk of moving to a new substage. That is why we speak of 'towards' a new substage and not 'until' a new substage.
- **At risk of progression**: If the patient remains in the same substage A after 6 months of management, Dysmobility must be considered at risk of progression.
- **Stable**: If the patient remains in the same substage A, after 12 months of management, Dysmobility should be considered stable.
- **Regression**: If the patient shows signs of improvement after 6 months of management, it can be considered that Dysmobility is in regression.

Patients in Substage B

For patients in substage B, three phases are considered:

- **In Progression**: During the first 12 months after diagnosis, Dysmobility should be considered progressing to the next stage.
- **At risk of progression**: If the patient remains in the same substage B after 12 months of management, Dysmobility is considered at risk of progression.

Table 5.1 Stability of Dysmobility

	Time of management		
Substage	0–6 months	6–12 months	>12 months
A	In progression	At risk of progression or in regression	Stable
B	In progression		At risk of progression or in regression

Based on Dinamarca Montecinos JL. De la Inmovilidad a la Dismovilidad en Geriatría. Ediciones de la Sociedad Chilena de Psicogeriatría, Santiago, Chile, 2004 [2]

– **In regression**: If the patient shows signs of improvement after 12 months of management, Dysmobility can be considered in regression.

Keynote: Only patients in substage A may be considered to have 'stable' Dysmobility, and only if they maintain strict management and supervision.

Stability is summarised in Table 5.1.

References

1. Dinamarca-Montecinos JL. Dysmobility in geriatrics. A decade defining a clinical concept. Bol Hosp Vina del Mar, 2012 68(2):15–19.
2. Dinamarca Montecinos JL. De la Inmovilidad a la Dismovilidad en Geriatría. Santiago: Ediciones de la Sociedad Chilena de Psicogeriatría; 2004.

Application of the Triaxial Diagnosis Method

6

How to Use the Triaxial Diagnostic Method

Dysmobility does not include a mere name change of a classic syndrome. It is a concept, and, as such, it entails a way of thinking and a way of acting.

Along with conceptual clarity, the triaxial diagnostic method is the first tool we need to correctly apply the concept of Dysmobility in geriatrics and achieve the best results for our patients.

In the next chapter, we carry out a review and description of the triaxial diagnosis process of Dysmobility in geriatrics.

Identification Process

Patient Identification

This may seem obvious. However, the diagnostic process is clinical and must have a written consequence, which must be carried out immediately. The first thing is to identify in writing the name and age of the patient, place and date of evaluation, name of the person (patient or caregiver) who provides the information, and name of the interviewer. For this, the card system is proposed, which can be reviewed at the end of this chapter.

J. L. Dinamarca-Montecinos, *Dysmobility in Geriatrics*, https://doi.org/10.1007/978-3-031-72716-0_6

Dysmobility Identification

Before applying the triaxial method, it is essential to objectify the existence of the syndrome, to avoid both underdiagnosis and overdiagnosis.

To objectify the presence or absence of Dysmobility, start asking the patient:

- Do you (or if the patient cannot answer, the interviewer can ask the caregiver, or if there is no caregiver, the interviewer can record his own perspective about the patient) have any discomfort or difficulty of any origin, when making any movement with any part of your body and/or when moving from one place to another?
- Do you (same as the previous question) have any inability, of any origin, to make any movement with any part of your body and/or to move from one place to another?

Comments

The first question seeks to account for symptomatic aspects, while the second is mainly about signs.

It should be emphasised that discomfort, difficulties, or impossibilities *can be of any origin. It must not* be articular or of origin in the musculoskeletal system. It can be vascular, respiratory, psychological, or even environmental. It could be, for example, that the patient could not travel from his home to the nearest health centre by his own means, due to environmental barriers that have become insurmountable with the means available to him. If so, the first question should be answered 'yes'.

It is also important to consider that the magnitude of the symptoms *does not matter*. It can be something as seemingly small as an eyelid tremor. This should lead to answering 'yes' to the first question, since it represents a difficulty when carrying out the normal movement of a part of the body, the eyelid.

These questions should always be asked, even if there is an obvious condition of Dysmobility, as they allow us to understand the degree of awareness of the patient's illness and/or his/her caregivers.

If the answer is 'no' to one or another question, but there is evidence of the presence of the syndrome, the interviewer will know that he or she will not be able to fully rely on the following answers and must have support from caregivers to obtain the best information.

Finally, if the answer is 'no' to both questions, the patient does not have Dysmobility, and it is not appropriate to implement the triaxial diagnostic process.

If the answer is 'yes', even in only one of the questions, the evaluation continues, applying The Triaxial Method of Diagnosis of Dysmobility.

Triaxial Method of Diagnosis of Dysmobility

Axis 1. Evolution Time

The time of evolution is evaluated by asking the patient (or if the patient cannot answer, the interviewer can ask the caregiver, or if there is no caregiver, the interviewer can record his own perspective about the patient) about both the symptoms and signs of mobility disorders:

- **How long have you had mobility problems?**

Comments

The objective of this question is to establish whether the mobility problems began more than a year ago or less than a year ago.

In the first case, we will be facing an Old Dysmobility and, in the second, a Recent Dysmobility.

The implications of this response are in terms of prognosis and treatment. The more time that has passed, the chances of recovery decrease, and the risk of complications and sequelae increases, making the therapeutic challenge greater.

Axis 2. Speed of Presentation

The question that should be asked of the patient and/or his or her caregiver is the following:

- **Did these mobility problems start slowly or rather abruptly?**

Comments

The objective of this question is to establish whether Dysmobility is Acute or Slow.

Although it is usually easy to answer this question, it may happen that the patient and/or his or her caregiver are not able to establish a form of presentation. It may also happen that they cannot decide on both alternatives. If so, a second question should be asked:

- **Tell me about how mobility problems began.**

To facilitate understanding of the objective of the question by the patient and/or caregiver, the evolution graphs of both types of Dysmobility can be presented (see Graphics 1 and 2 in Chap. 4).

The objective of this question is to have data that guides regarding possible aetiologies.

With the information provided, it will be up to the clinician to define the form of presentation of Dysmobility.

Axis 3: D-STAGING

Once the time of evolution and the speed of presentation have been established, the staging of the Dysmobility must be carried out.

We will begin by remembering the definition of D-STAGING and describing its characteristics.

What Is D-STAGING?

- It is a dynamic continuum identification system of stages of Dysmobility, with clinical, therapeutic, prognostic, and scientific objectives.
- It allows to identify 5 stages of Dysmobility, with 2 substages each. That is, it consists of 10 substages.
- It was built for use on the population aged 60 or over and with motor disorders.
- It is a hetero-applied system; if the patient is not able to respond, the information can be obtained or compared with the main caregiver.
- It must be applied by personnel with competencies in geriatrics.
- It requires brief prior training.

Applying D-STAGING

First Question: Identification of the Usual Motor Segment

It seeks to roughly determine the motor stage in which the patient is, that is, whether he or she spends more time standing (segment 1), sitting (segment 2), or lying down (segment 3).

- **On average, during the past month, does the patient spend most of the day standing, sitting, or lying down?**

Comments

It is important to note that D-STAGING seeks to determine what the patient does, not what the patient is capable to do but do not do:

  – If a patient spends most of the day lying down but 'would be able to walk', this patient will be in motor segment 3 (in bed), not 1 (standing).
  – If a patient spends most of the day sitting but 'is capable' of spending most of the day walking, it is appropriate to classify within the stages of sitting (segment 2), not standing (segment 1).

This should be made clear to the interviewee to avoid false staging: The question is about what the patient DOES, NOT what the patient 'WOULD BE ABLE TO DO'.

Regarding 'most of the day' part of the question, this is defined as 'the usual period of greatest activity of the person from the moment they wake up until they fall asleep'.

They are usually between 8 and 12 h, usually during daylight hours.

However, there are people who carry out nocturnal activities and sleep during the day.

The concept is 'during the patient's usual period of activity'.

In the case of patients with inversion of the sleep-wake cycle, this meaning is not valid, and it is assumed that 'most of the day' is daytime.

It is interesting to note that both the question and the answer may surprise: Many self-sufficient people spend most of their day sitting. Therefore, if they have any motor symptoms, they could be considered carriers of stage 2-A Dysmobility. This would correspond to a clinical definition of 'sedentary lifestyle': spending most of the day in a sitting position.

Second Question and Following

After determining the usual motor segment, we seek to define the corresponding substage, asking about its characterisation. Depending on the usual motor segment, there will be one or more questions to ask to achieve this.

For patients spending most of the day on their feet

- **Do you need any type of help from another person, technical help, or support with any element to walk?**
  - If the answer is 'no', the patient will classify 1-A.
  - If the answer is 'yes', the patient will classify 1-B.

Comments

The support elements can be anything: walls, furniture, canes, other people, etc. Many patients will say that they do not need a cane, but the reality is that they need to lean on the furniture in their home to be able to walk.

Patients in substage 1-B tend quickly to develop the habit of sitting most of the day. Monitor the amount of time the patient spends sitting, and alert him or her to the risk of spending more time sitting.

For patients spending most of the day sitting

- **Is the patient able to sit and stand up alone, without help from anyone?**
  - If the answer is yes, the patient will classify 2-A.
  - If the answer is no, the patient will classify 2-B.

Comments

Patients in substage 2-B are at greater risk of remaining bedridden.

Many times, substage 2-B accounts for patients who, if not lifted by their caregivers, would spend the entire day in bed. This reflects, on the one hand, the importance of caregivers and, on the other, the importance of removing patients from their beds who, with a simple change in position, go from a profound stage of Dysmobility to a much less compromising one.

For patients spending most of the day in bed

- **Does he/she get out of bed on his/her own?** (E.g. to the bathroom or to take out food)
  - Yes: 3-A
- **No: Do the patient sit on the edge of the bed without help?**
  - Yes: 3-B
- **No: Does the patient move on his/her own in bed, changing positions and turning without help?**
  - Yes: 4-A
- **No: Does the patient move on his/her own in bed but need help to turn?**
  - Yes: 4-B
- **No: Can the patient make himself/herself understood in some way by the people who care for him/her?**
  - Yes: 5-A
  - No: 5-B

Comments

The staging of life-in-bed (we will use 'bedridden' from here) (substages 3-A to 5-B) is based on the risks of associated complications.

Among them, the risk of pressure injuries stands out, which increases exponentially with the difficulty of turning, changing position by one's own means and/or warning of possible difficulties.

Other important complications are accelerated sarcopenia, which itself appears when the patient becomes bedridden, and thromboembolic disease of the deep venous system of the lower extremities.

Research on Dysmobility 7

Introduction

This chapter presents the results of a search of publications for the Spanish terms 'Dismovilidad' (Dysmobility) and 'ETADI' (D-STAGING, Etapificación de la Dismovilidad by its acronym in Spanish), in the repositories Google Scholar, LILACS, REDALYC, and SciELO, between the years 2004 and 2024. Publications in indexed scientific journals, theses to obtain an academic degree, clinical guidelines, and academic books were selected.

Subsequently, the main responses and trends are summarised, and future lines of research are proposed.

Likewise, the reader is warned of the main risks of research in this area.

One hundred thirty-six publications were found.

One hundred twelve were excluded due to:

- Use of the term 'Dysmobility' as a synonym for 'immobility'
- Use of the term 'Dysmobility' without reference to any concept
- Use of D-Staging as a system to perform sampling
- Publications made by the same author

J. L. Dinamarca-Montecinos, *Dysmobility in Geriatrics*,
https://doi.org/10.1007/978-3-031-72716-0_7

The remaining 24 publications were classified into the following five subgroups:

(a) **Conceptual**
Mainly related to the concept of Dysmobility in geriatrics, discussing the definition, the triaxial method, or other aspects.
(b) **Comparisons**
Mainly, they compare D-STAGING with other measurement methods, mostly functionality and activities of daily living scales.
(c) **Clinical-epidemiological**
Mainly, they use D-STAGING to objectify the clinical evolution of groups of patients and/or compare groups of subjects looking for patterns based on the substages of D-STAGING to define etiological, therapeutic, and prognostic aspects.
(d) **Academics (scholarly activity or thesis)**
They use the concept of Dysmobility in research associated with the achievement of an academic or professional degree, as part of the last academic year at a university.
(e) **Public policies**
They propose the concept of Dysmobility in the assessment of older people at various levels of health care through documents generated by experts and national references at the Ministerial level.

The main aspects of each publication are summarised below.

Research on Dysmobility

Conceptual

Luna, L. Geriatric syndromes compromise the autonomy and functionality of older adults. In: The health of older adults, a shared vision. Pan American Health Organization, 2nd Ed, 2011. Chapter 9, immobility syndrome, pp. 193–197. ISBN 978-92-75-33250-4.

The chapter is dedicated to several geriatric syndromes, including immobility. The author proposes changing the concept to 'Dysmobility' exposing the definition and associated concepts. In addition, she complements this with practical suggestions to consider when caring for patients with deep-stage Dysmobility [1].

Reyes Álvarez Pedro Luis. General procedures for the delivery of resources to incontinent and bedridden patients, an imperative appreciation. Rev. Medical Sciences. 2018 Feb;22(1):29–37.

In this work, a review of the document 'Procedure for the sale of resources to bedridden, incontinent and bedridden people' is carried out. This is a joint instruction (03/93/PI) of the Ministry of Health of Cuba and the Ministry of Internal Trade. It is proposed to stop using the term 'prostration', using instead the concept of Dysmobility, its definition, and the triaxial diagnostic system to improve understanding by patients, caregivers, and authorities and optimise both the implementation and monitoring of the resources delivered [2].

Reyes Álvarez, Pedro Luis. Immobility and prostration or Dysmobility and bedding? Scientific Rev. med. Pinar Rio; 21(1):2–3, Jan.-Feb. 2017.

The importance of objectifying or definitively changing the concepts of 'immobility' and 'prostration' for 'Dysmobility' and 'bedding' is discussed, to optimise the quality of clinical management in general [3].

The proposal of using a new meaning for the term 'bedding' (as a simile of 'lying-in-bed') is interesting.

González Farfán ME. J. Dinamarca Immobility Syndrome Scale, useful but incomplete tool. Rev. Hered Rehab. 2016;1:83–84.

D-STAGING is compared with the Red Cross Physical Disability Scale, finding that some constructs or stages could be relatively similar. Some shortcomings are evident in the understanding and application of D-STAGING [4].

González MLN. Immobilization syndrome in the elderly. Rev. Med Cos Cen. 2015;72(616):551–555.

Definitions of immobilization or immobility syndrome are summarised, including the definition of Dysmobility and proposing its use. However, the use of the term 'immobilization' is maintained throughout the article, although it is recognised that the absence of movement does not really exist [5].

Comparatives

Martínez J, Bravo S, Chipia J. Association between functional status and Dysmobility in hospitalized geriatric patients. Community and Health 2019, 17(2):27–37.

In this study, 143 patients hospitalised at the San Isidro Labrador Geriatric Clinic Hospital in the period January–December 2014 were selected, comparing D-STAGING with the FIM and Modified Rankin scales. A significant association was found between the levels of Dysmobility, the stages of these scales, and age: the older the patients, the worse the mobility levels according to D-STAGING and functionality according to FIM and Rankin. No association was found between sex and stages of Dysmobility [6].

Clinical

Soto Fernández O, Barrios Casas S. Characterization of health, dependency, immobility, and risk of pressure ulcers of patients admitted to the home care program. Science Ill; 18(3):61–72, 2012.

In this work, D-STAGING was used to describe the frequency of anatomical and functional complications in a group of patients living in their own homes, in the city of Puerto Montt, Chile. A direct relationship was established between the depth of Dysmobility and the level of dependency and between the depth of Dysmobility and the risk of pressure injuries [7].

von Mühlenbrock F, Gómez R, González V, Rojas A, Vargas G, von Mühlenbrock P. Prevalence of Depression in patients over 60 years of age hospitalized in the Internal Medicine Service of the Military Hospital of Santiago. Chilean Journal of Neuropsychiatry, 2011, 49(4):331–337.

The association of D-STAGING with depression is evaluated in an elderly population hospitalised in an internal medicine service. A value close to statistical significance (but not significant) was calculated. There was an association between deeper Dysmobility and diagnosis of depression [8].

Epidemiological

Becerra Hoebel V, Becerra Hoebel E, Tiznado Retamal J. Prevalence of anemia in the dismobile elderly patient at the Nueva Aurora Clinic. Bol. Hosp. Viña del Mar 2009, 65(3/4): 104–109.

Describes a local population in the city of Viña del Mar, Chile; using D-STAGING to differentiate home patients and comparing levels of Dysmobility with the frequency of anaemia. It was found that both the frequency and severity of anaemia increased with increasing depth of Dysmobility ($p < 0.005$) [9].

Becerra Hoebel V, Becerra Hoebel E, Tiznado Retamal J. Profile of chronic pathology of dismobile older adults at the Nueva Aurora Clinic. Bol. Hosp. Viña del Mar 2009; 65(3/4): 110–117.

This work describes that the most frequent causes of Dysmobility in a home program in Chile were strokes and organic brain damage [10].

Zaldívar Suárez N, Saborit Oliva Y, Elías Postigo O, Collejo Rosabal Y, Robles Ortiz J. Dysmobility syndrome in the "Lidia Doce" nursing home. Multimed (Granma); 26(4): e2171, Jul.-Aug. 2022.

This work describes a pattern that relates age between 80 and 90 years with Dysmobility in stage 1, and over 90 years with Dysmobility in stage 3, in an institutionalised population in Granma, Cuba [11].

Ulloa Chávez O, Martínez Muñoz L, Hernández Ferreras K, Fernández Correa L. Immobility syndrome in older adults at the Bernardo Posse Polyclinic in the San Miguel del Padrón municipality. Gac Méd Espirit. 2019; 21(3):30–39.

One hundred seventy-one older adults from a polyclinic in Cuba are characterised according to whether the Dysmobility was acute or slow. No reference is made to either the definition of Dysmobility or the triaxial method, and, throughout the article, only immobility syndrome is mentioned. Approximately two-thirds of the sample presented slow Dysmobility, the remaining third, acute [12].

Academics (Scholarly Activity or Thesis)

Valverde Supo LE. Evaluation of Dysmobility syndrome upon admission and discharge in older adults hospitalised in the Department of Medicine of the Honorio Delgado Espinoza General Hospital of Arequipa, in January and February 2019. Repository of the Universidad San Agustín de Arequipa, Peru 2019.

Two hundred eighteen patients over 60 years were studied, all of them admitted to the Department of Medicine of the Honorio Delgado Espinoza General Hospital in Arequipa, Peru, with D-STAGING applied at admission and discharge. It was established that, with older age, the depth of Dysmobility upon admission was greater, significantly increasing the frequency of bedridden among patients over 80 years of age. Likewise, there were no differences between sexes in this parameter. It was also shown that hospitalization significantly influenced the mobility of patients, reducing it. The more profound the Dysmobility at admission, the worse the impact of hospitalization on the patients' motor capacity [13].

Quiroga Ortiz N. Risk factors for Dysmobility Syndrome in older adults in the home Daniel Álvarez Sánchez. Repository of the National University of Loja, Ecuador, 2015.

Prospective study in which a population of 50 people living in care homes is classified, characterizing the diseases that generate the risk of Dysmobility. A 56% frequency of the syndrome was found, with the most frequent stages being those of sitting. The deeper stages of Dysmobility were associated with malnutrition, multimorbidity, and older ages; stage 2B presented a higher frequency of dysthymia/depression. The most prevalent associated diseases in this group were urinary incontinence, osteoarthritis, high blood pressure, rheumatoid arthritis, dementia, type 2 diabetes mellitus, and heart disease [14].

Rodríguez PC, Pauta DV. Relationship between Dysmobility and the fear of falling with Geronte's family factors. Digital repository, National University of Loja, Ecuador.

The cross-sectional correlational study, as part of the macro-project 'Quality of Life in the elderly, zone 7 of Ecuador', with stratified random sampling of 1146 subjects aged 65 or older out of a universe of 99,563.

The objective was to establish if there was a relationship between family dysfunction, Dysmobility, and fear of falling. Family functionality was measured with the FF-SIL test, Dysmobility was staged with D-STAGING, and fear of falling was assessed using the FES-I test. Dysmobility was associated with a greater fear of falling (OR 1.52; $p < 0.05$) and a greater presence of family dysfunction (OR 1.49, $p < 0.05$) [15].

Navarrete Vilca T. Functional assessment and staging of Dysmobility in older adults upon hospital admission to a specialized Geriatric Clinic of social security in EsSalud in Lima, Peru, 2013. Repository of the Peruvian University of Applied Sciences, Lima 2013.

In this retrospective study with 180 patients acutely hospitalised in a geriatrics service, it is established that there is a strong association between staging with D-STAGING and the level of functionality at admission measured with the Katz index. The higher the level of independence, according to the categorised Katz index, the greater the probability of having Dysmobility corresponding to stages 1–2, even considering adjustment for other relevant covariates. Likewise, the greater the dependency, the correlation with Dysmobility in stages of bed rest is greater [16].

Aravena Romero M, Grangey Trujillo F. Incidence of burnout syndrome in caregivers of older adults with severe dependency or Dysmobility at the San José Nursing Home in the commune of Recoleta. Repository of the Silva Henríquez Catholic University, Faculty of Health Sciences, Chile 2017.

In this work, a sample of 28 older adults residing in a long-term institution is characterised, evaluating the correlation between the level of Dysmobility (measured with D-STAGING) and functionality (measured with Barthel), with caregiver overload (measured with Maslach Burnout Inventory). Dysmobility in the sitting stage is described in almost half of the population studied and a weak correlation of stage 2B with greater caregiver stress [17].

Letelier Matisen R, Yáñez Yáñez R. Determination of the degree of functional dependence of patients in the Geriatrics Service of the Doctor Lautaro Navarro Avaria Regional Hospital in the city of Punta Arenas through the application of the Functional Independence Measure (FIM) and its relationship with the Dysmobility Syndrome. Repository of the University of Magallanes, Chile, 2009.

A comparative study with 26 patients in which D-STAGING is correlated with FIM, establishing that functional dependence measured with FIM and depth of Dysmobility measured with D-STAGING are directly proportional: The greater the depth of Dysmobility, the greater the motor, cognitive, and functional dependence. When separating stages into substages, D-STAGING substages B were related to less functional and cognitive independence, compared to substages A, which had greater functional and cognitive independence [18].

Astargo C, Ayala K, Droguett C, González S, Martínez M, Martínez Y. Adaptability in families with bedridden older adults, from the home program of two health centers in Valparaíso. Theses Repository of the University of Valparaíso, Chile, 2008.

The characteristics of the families caring for 33 bedridden elderly people belonging to two home programs are described, using the complete concept of Dysmobility. Similarly, the characteristics of the sample according to D-STAGING are described.

About 80% of caregivers are 50 years old or older (nearly 45% are 60 years old or older, and about 33% are between 50 and 60 years old). Fifty-two percent of the care network for these patients is extended family, and 42% is nuclear family. When nuclear family, in 24% the main caregiver is the couple and in 55% a child of the patient (72% daughter and 28% son).

The age of the bedridden patients was over 75 years in 72.7%; the percentages doubled every 10 years from the age of 60. At older ages, there is a clear predominance of women.

The patients all had Dysmobility in the bedridden phase (3-A onwards), the most frequent being stages 4 (57.6%) and 5 (30.3%), with a predominance of Slow Dysmobility (58%) and Old Dysmobility (88%).

There was no relationship between the time of evolution of Dysmobility and the degree of flexibility of the family [19].

Public Policies

Various authors. Undersecretary of Public Health Disease, Prevention, and Control Division. Life Cycle Department, National Office of Comprehensive Health for Older People 2022, Ministry of Health of Chile. Nursing Manual: Role of Gerontogeriatric Nursing in the Continuing Care of the Elderly. Chapter 8, nursing care in ELEAM. Chapter 14, nursing care in older people with Dysmobility syndrome.

The reconceptualization of immobility syndrome as Dysmobility syndrome is made explicit. The concepts of classification of Dysmobility are provided according to its form of installation, time of evolution, and stage in which it is found, emphasizing that the form of installation allows differentiating aetiologies, evolution, prognosis, and different treatments. They highlight as well that staging with D-STAGING enables the user to define the level of care, therapeutic and preventative measures, and having a reference standard of the effectiveness of the measures implemented so that a functional and vital prognosis can be established. The triaxial method is proposed to assess elderly patients at different levels of care by nursing professionals. It is proposed that nursing professionals who care for elderly people with disabilities use the concept of Dismobility [20].

Azócar Valenzuela MJ, Mohor Valentino C, Rioja Ponce R, Vargas Leyton M. Quality standards for long-stay establishments for older adults. Protocols of the National Service for the Elderly, Chile 2016. SENAMA Editions, ISBN: 978-956-8846-10-7.

The concept of Dysmobility and the triaxial diagnostic method (including D-STAGING) are integrated into the clinical management of older people who require care in long-stay institutions in the State of Chile [21].

Various authors. Technical health standard for the comprehensive health care of older adults. NTS-207 of 2023 of the Ministry of Health of Peru.

Among the fundamental definitions of the document, the definition of Dysmobility is included, with the objective of 'contributing to the comprehensive care of older adults, as well as their functional capacity, well-being, dignity and quality of life in the country' [22].

Comments

Both the definition of Dysmobility and the triaxial diagnostic method, as well as the concept of continuous motor, are recommended for a reconceptualisation of the immobility syndrome. Its active use is proposed in the clinic and in health policies, to facilitate its programming, implementation, and monitoring. The older concepts of 'immobility' and 'prostration' are progressively understood as parts of the final stages of Dysmobility [1–3, 19–22].

D-STAGING has a good correlation with other instruments, particularly those that measure disability and risks of complications associated with Dysmobility (Red Cross Physical Disability Scale, FIM, modified Rankin, Katz index, Braden-Bergstrom scale, and GNEAUPP) [4, 6, 7, 16, 18].

Difficulties persist when applying D-STAGING, with errors being made that are mostly due to the use of the instrument alone, without a correct understanding of the definition and without the triaxial diagnosis method [5, 6].

The relationship between stages of Dysmobility and the sex of the patients seems to depend on the time of evolution and depth of Dysmobility: In acute Dysmobility and patients up to stage 2, no relationship has been found [6, 7, 13], while in patients with old and profound Dysmobility, there is a predominance of women [19].

It has been found that Slow Dysmobility is more common than acute Dysmobility; the ratio would be 2:1 [12, 19].

Some nosological entities have been indicated as producing Dysmobility in general and others associated with some stages. Dysmobility in deep stages of displacement has been associated with stroke and neurocognitive disorder [10].

Several studies describe significant associations, directly proportional, between the depth of Dysmobility and the following:

- Age of patients [6, 11],
- Risk of pressure injuries [7, 13].
- Frequency and severity of anaemia [9].
- Worse motor capacity after hospitalisation for an acute cause [13].
- There could be a relationship between the stages of Dysmobility and the risk of suffering from depression [8, 14].

According to stages:

- Stage 2-B of Slow Dysmobility is related to a greater frequency of depression [14].
- Stage 2-B correlates with greater caregiver burden [17].
- The stages of placement (3-A onwards) are associated with membership in home programs [19].
- Stage 4 was the most frequent in a study of home patients [19].

Risks of Research with Dysmobility

The non-use, underuse, or inadequate use of the Dysmobility-associated concepts: definition, concept of continuous motor, and triaxial method.

The incomplete use of the concept of Dysmobility or its non-integrative atomisation (e.g. using D-STAGING as a synonym for

Dysmobility) is a common error that can lead to inadequate results in research.

A thorough understanding of the concept of motor continuum and the definition of Dysmobility is essential along with the correct application of the triaxial method, including D-STAGING.

Future of Research with Dysmobility

Currently, there are many clinical publications that refer to Dysmobility as a simple synonym for the old immobility, inappropriately using the concept of Dysmobility. One of the objectives that must be set is the correct use of these concepts in the clinical setting.

An interesting step will be to carry out clinical and organisational studies. Considering 'organisational' in both senses: how the implementation of the concept of Dysmobility impacts organisational indicators in health and how Dysmobility concepts, models, and theoretical frameworks can be better implemented, using specific tools [23, 24].

The concept of Dysmobility (definition, triaxial method, and staging) must be used in an appropriate and complementary manner, avoiding the use of Dysmobility as a synonym for 'immobility'. It must be remembered that 'immobility' is a term, while Dysmobility is a concept.

In this aspect, the conceptual map for the Dysmobility researcher should consider the following 'grid' (Table 7.1).

In this grid, the *X* axis represents time (form of presentation and time of evolution at the time of diagnosis), and the *Y* axis represents the depth of Dysmobility (according to staging with D-STAGING).

The variables can be those that the researcher decides: risk of depression, caregiver overload, functional prognosis, response to a rehabilitation protocol, vital risk, motor manifestations in a particular type of nosological entity (hip fractures, ischemic stroke, etc.) in a specific type of Dysmobility, and even in a single stage, to give some examples.

Table 7.1 Conceptual map for the Dysmobility researcher

		Time (Form of presentation and time of evolution)		
		SOD (slow old Dysmobility)	ARD (acute recent Dysmobility)	AOD (acute old Dysmobility)
DEEP (D-STAGING)	1-A			
	1-B			
	2-A			
	2-B			
	3-A			
	3-B			
	4-A			
	4-B			
	5-A			
	5-B			

The establishment of diagnostic-therapeutic units is a great challenge, seeking the associations and relationships that occur between the different types and stages of Dysmobility and specific nosological entities, such as depression.

Discomfort, difficulties, and/or impossibilities of any organ or system, including those not involved in locomotion, should be considered part of the dismobilising process and integrated into the investigation. In fact, if we carefully consider the definition of Dysmobility, we will find that they are very common among older people. Just to name a few examples, we have disorders of the temporomandibular joint, swallowing, intestinal transit, and arrhythmias.

In the clinical setting, there is the possibility of working on characterization according to level of care, risk and prognosis profiles, social profiles, and psychological profiles, opening the possibility of carrying out research in Dysmobility for all health-related professions.

In addition to the clinical setting, the concept of Dysmobility (definition, triaxial method, and staging) is useful in the organizational setting. This, then, allows us to limit and homogenise resource implementation criteria and to more closely compare the results obtained. In this way, the inclusion of the concept of Dysmobility in quality systems is an interesting area of research.

It is very likely that movement problems are directly related to the different forms of aging. Considering all systems in the concept of Dysmobility, including, for example, molecular ones, can lead us to unsuspected keys.

References

1. Luna L. Geriatric syndromes compromise the autonomy and functionality of older adults. The health of older adults, a shared vision. In: Chapter 9: Immobility syndrome. 2nd ed. Pan American Health Organization; 2011. p. 193–7. https://iris.paho.org/handle/10665.2/51598.
2. Luis RÁP. General procedures for the delivery of resources to incontinent and bedridden patients, an imperative appreciation. Rev Med Sci. 2018;22(1):29–37. http://scielo.sld.cu/scielo.php?script=sci_arttext&pid=S1561319420180001000006&lng=es.
3. Álvarez R, Luis P. Immobility and prostration or Dysmobility and bedding? Sci Rev med Pinar Rio. 2017;21(1):2–3.
4. González Farfán MEJ. Dinamarca immobility syndrome scale, useful but incomplete tool. Rev Hered Rehab. 2016;1:83–4.
5. González MLN. Immobilization syndrome in the elderly. Rev Med Cos Cen. 2015;72(616):551–5.
6. Martínez J, Bravo S, Chipia J. Association between functional status and Dysmobility in hospitalized geriatric patients. Community Health. 2019;17(2):27–37.
7. Soto Fernández O, Barrios CS. Characterization of health, dependency, immobility, and risk of pressure ulcers of patients admitted to the home care program. Sci ill. 2012;18(3):61–72.
8. von Mühlenbrock F, Gómez R, González V, Rojas A, Vargas G, von Mühlenbrock P. Prevalence of depression in patients over 60 years of age hospitalized in the Internal Medicine Service of the Military Hospital of Santiago. Chilean J Neuropsychiatry. 2011;49(4):331–7.
9. Becerra Hoebel V, Becerra Hoebel E, Tiznado RJ. Prevalence of anemia in the dismobile elderly patient at the Nueva Aurora Clinic. Bol Hosp Viña del Mar. 2009;65(3/4):104–9.
10. Becerra Hoebel V, Becerra Hoebel E, Tiznado RJ. Profile of chronic pathology of dismobile older adults at the Nueva Aurora Clinic. Bol Hosp Viña del Mar. 2009;65(3/4):110–7.
11. Zaldívar Suárez N, Saborit Oliva Y, Elías Postigo O, Collejo Rosabal Y, Robles OJ. Dysmobility syndrome in the "Lidia Doce" nursing home. Multimed (Granma). 2022;26(4):e2171.

12. Ulloa Chávez O, Martínez Muñoz L, Hernández Ferreras K, Fernández CL. Immobility syndrome in older adults at the Bernardo posse polyclinic in the San Miguel del Padrón municipality. Gac Méd Espirit. 2019;21(3):30–9. http://scielo.sld.cu/scielo.php?script=sci_arttext&pid=S1608-89212019000300030&lng=es.
13. Valverde Supo LE. Evaluation of Dysmobility syndrome upon admission and discharge in older adults hospitalized in the Department of Medicine of the Honorio Delgado Espinoza general Hospital of Arequipa, in January and February 2019. Arequipa: Universidad San Agustín de Arequipa; 2019. https://repositorio.unsa.edu.pe/server/api/core/bitstreams/9ef79325-130e-463a-a733-5b011f2b9037/content.
14. Quiroga ON. Risk factors for Dysmobility syndrome in older adults in the home Daniel Álvarez Sánchez. Loja: National University of Loja; 2015. https://dspace.unl.edu.ec/jspui/bitstream/123456789/13497/1/TESIS%20IMPRIMIR%20PRESENTAR%20imp.pdf.
15. Rodríguez PC, Pauta DV. Relationship between Dysmobility and the fear of falling with Geronte's family factors. Loja: National University of Loja; 2017. https://dspace.unl.edu.ec/jspui/handle/123456789/18387.
16. Navarrete VT. Functional assessment and staging of Dysmobility in older adults upon hospital admission to a specialized geriatric clinic of social security in Essalud in Lima, Peru, 2013. Lima: Peruvian University of Applied Sciences; 2013. https://repositorioacademico.upc.edu.pe/bitstream/handle/10757/621836/NAVARRETE_VT.pdf?sequence=5.
17. Aravena Romero M, Grangey TF. Incidence of burnout syndrome in caregivers of older adults with severe dependency or Dysmobility at the San José nursing home in the commune of Recoleta. Santiago: Silva Henríquez Catholic University; 2017. http://repositorio.ucsh.cl/xmlui/bitstream/handle/ucsh/1251/121185.pdf?sequence=1&isAllowed=y.
18. Letelier Matisen R, Yáñez R. Determination of the degree of functional dependence of patients in the geriatrics Service of the Doctor Lautaro Navarro Avaria Regional Hospital in the city of Punta Arenas through the application of the functional Independence measure (MIF) and its relationship with the Dysmobility syndrome. Punta Arenas: University of Magallanes; 2009. http://www.umag.cl/biblioteca/tesis/letelier_matisen_2009.pdf.
19. Astargo C, Ayala K, Droguett C, González S, Martínez M, Martínez Y. Adaptability in families with bedridden older adults, from the home program of two health centers in Valparaíso. Valparaíso: University of Valparaíso; 2008. https://repositoriobibliotecas.uv.cl/serveruv/api/core/bitstreams/116ccb1d-5130-472b-9120-ce42eb2c1172/content.
20. Various Authors. Undersecretary of Public Health Disease, Prevention, and Control Division. Life Cycle Department, National Office of Comprehensive Health for Older People 2022, Ministry of Health of Chile. Nursing Manual: Role of Gerontogeriatric Nursing in the Continuing Care of the Elderly. Chapter 8, nursing care in

ELEAM. Chapter 14, nursing care in older people with Disability syndrome. https://diprece.minsal.cl/wp-content/uploads/2023/11/26_07_23-ENFERMERIA-personas-mayores.pdf.
21. Azócar Valenzuela MJ, Mohor Valentino C, Rioja Ponce R, Vargas LM. Quality standards for long-stay establishments for older adults. Protocols of the National Service for the Elderly, Chile. SENAMA Editions; 2016.
22. Various Authors. Technical health standard for the comprehensive health care of older adults. NTS-207 of 2023 of the Ministry of Health of Peru. https://www.gob.pe/institucion/minsa/normas-legales/4557563-789-2023-minsa.
23. Nilsen P. Making sense of implementation theories, models and frameworks. Implement Sci. 2015;10:53. https://doi.org/10.1186/s13012-015-0242-0.
24. Bergström A, Ehrenberg A, Eldh A, et al. The use of the PARIHS framework in implementation research and practice—a citation analysis of the literature. Implement Sci. 2020;15:68. https://doi.org/10.1186/s13012-020-01003-0.

Clinical Cases 8

Introduction

In this chapter, we apply the triaxial diagnostic method of Dysmobility, and we propose a way of ordering concomitant diseases and the social care network and a way of organizing management.

Competencies

After applying the concepts of the book to resolve the cases in this chapter, the health-related professional should:

- Understand that the use of the concept of Dysmobility is part of their technical training.
- Understand that the use of the concept 'prostration' is not appropriate in health (see the note at the end of Chap. 3).
- Be able to carry out a general diagnostic approach through the application of D-STAGING.
- Propose contributions from his/her own specialty to the interdisciplinary management of patients with Dysmobility.

J. L. Dinamarca-Montecinos, *Dysmobility in Geriatrics*,
https://doi.org/10.1007/978-3-031-72716-0_8

The diagnosis and management process of the patient with Dysmobility must be carried out by addressing the following points:

1. **Diagnosis**:
   (a) Motor:
   - Presence/absence of Dysmobility
   - Form of presentation
   - Time of evolution
   - Staging

   (b) Diseases:
   - Base conditions and Aetiology of Dysmobility
   - Complications

   (c) Social environment:
   - Identify.
   - Describe.
2. **Management**:
   (a) Motor goals:
   - Set the level of care.
   - Prioritise care.
   - Determine the diseases that should be studied.

   (b) Objectives according to diseases:
   - Compensate/stabilise.
   - Determine presence/risks and prevent and/or implement treatment.

   (c) Social objectives
   - Include the social network (if existing) in the health work.
   - Form the social network (if not existing)
   - Stabilise the social network.

This is visualised through a Dysmobility map, which is presented in Table 8.1:

To complement the reading and compare the process of the following clinical cases, the reader can review Chap. 4 (Diagnosis of Dysmobility) particularly Table 8.2 (D-STAGING) and Chap. 6 (Application of the Triaxial Method).

Table 8.1 Dysmobility map

Level	Diagnosis	Management
Motor	**Form of presentation**	**Establish level of care**:
	Acute Dysmobility	Hospital, home
	Slow Dysmobility	Outpatient, home, community
	Time of evolution	**Establish priority of care and health team**:
	Recent Dysmobility	Start interdisciplinary rehabilitation as soon as possible
	Old Dysmobility	According to prognosis, expectations, and possibilities
	D-STAGING	**Establish level of care**
	Stage 1	Outpatient or community
	Stage 2	Outpatient or home
	Stages 3–5	Outpatient, domiciliary
	D-STAGING sub-phases:	**Establish general objectives**:
	Substage A	Avoid/slow progression, achieve regression
	Substage B	Return to better previous stage
Diseases	**Basal conditions**	**Define the main aetiology of Dysmobility**:
		To establish objectives: keep offset/stabilised
	Complications	**Establish objectives**:
		Existing complications: diagnose and treat
		Risk of complications: define and prevent
Social	**Existing social network**	**Establish objectives**:
		Describe, include, train, stabilise
	Not existing	**Establish objectives**:
		Describe the environment and form a social network

Table 8.2 Dysmobility map clinical case 1 (acute recent dysmobility)

Level	Diagnosis	Management
Motor	**Form of presentation** Acute Dysmobility	**Level of care**: Home (previous: emergency and hospital)
	Time of evolution Recent Dysmobility	**Priority in care**: Start interdisciplinary rehabilitation as soon as possible: Home training for caregivers Kinesiological and speech therapy rehabilitation for patient **Equipment**: Doctor, nurse, caregivers, kinesiologist, speech therapist
	D-STAGING Stages 3–5 **D-STAGING substages**: Substage B	**Level of care**: domiciliary **Set general objectives**: Avoid progression Return to the best previous stage Get out of bed (**get out of bed!!**) Take to stage 2-B to maintain trunk control and respiratory and circulatory capacities

Diseases	**Basal conditions**	**Define the main aetiology of Dysmobility**: Cardioembolic stroke of the right Sylvian valley, due to intermittent atrial fibrillation **Objectives**: Avoid new stroke Compensate heart rate Start anticoagulation
	Complications	**Existing**: **search, study, and treat** – Pharyngeal phase dysphagia – Left hemineglect – Left facial, brachial and crural hemiparesis – Drowsiness **Risk**: prevent – Depression
Social	**Existing social network**	**Describe** Four children, all willing to take care of her **Include** Generation of care shift calendar Definition of roles and primary caregiver Definition of decision-making instance **Train** Delivery of graphic material on underlying diseases **Stabilise** Emotional support and health help Definition of therapeutic objectives

Case 1: Acute Recent Dysmobility

Female, 87 years old, previously self-employed, homeowner, with Barthel 100 1 month ago. She suffered a right Silviano valley stroke 21 days ago. In the emergency room, intermittent atrial fibrillation was observed. Thrombolysis is performed. She was hospitalised and began subcutaneous thromboprophylaxis and interdisciplinary management of pharyngeal phase dysphagia, hemineglect, and left facial, brachial, and femoral hemiparesis. After 20 days, a gastrostomy is performed, enteral feeding is started, and the patient is referred to home, where the diagnostic process for Dysmobility is carried out.

Phase 1: Motor Diagnosis

(a) Identification of motor alteration:
- Do you (or the patient in your care) have any discomfort or difficulty of any origin, when making any movement with any part of your body and/or when moving from one place to another? YES
- Do you (or the patient in your care) have any inability, of any origin, to make any movement with any part of your body and/or to move from one place to another? YES

(b) Triaxial method of diagnosis of Dysmobility

Axis 1. Form of presentation:

- Did these mobility problems start slowly or rather abruptly? Abrupt, sharp.

Axis 2. Evolution time:

- How long have you/the patient in your care had mobility problems? 21 days

Axis 3: D-STAGING
First question: identification of the usual motor segment.

- On average, during the past month, does the patient spend most of the day standing, sitting, or lying down? Lying down in bed

Next:

If the patient spends most of the day in bed:

- Does the patient get out of bed on his own (e.g. to the bathroom or to take out food)?
- No: Does the patient sit on the edge of the bed without help?
- No: Does the patient move on his own in bed, change positions, and turn without help?
- No: Does the patient move around in bed on his own but need help turning?
- Yes: 4-B.

The Dysmobility map for clinical case 1 can be reviewed in Table 8.2.

Case 2: Acute Old Dysmobility

Male, 65 years old, executive in a marketing company, actively working. Three years ago, he suffered septic arthritis of the right hip, treated by traumatology with surgical cleansing and antibiotics, evolving well from the infection, but with rapid and progressive loss of joint function. In fact, he says that 'after the infection, my right hip was never completely fine'. He goes to an outpatient medical consultation due to pain that has been going on for a year and a half, in the right groin. He states that he has not been able to flex his hip for 2 and a half years. He has no problems standing statically, but when walking he develops left inguinal pain. When he sits down, he must do so in a chair with foot support, and it is very difficult for him to get up, although he can do it alone. Because of this, it is already very difficult for him to drive vehicles, which is important in the field in which he works. On the other hand, he gets very tired because he cannot rest sitting almost anywhere, so he prefers to walk on his feet all day.

The physical examination showed complete loss of the joint ranges of the right hip, with inguinal pain associated with muscle contractures, especially right extensor and adductor muscle atrophy, with exquisite pain on inguinal palpation. The anteroposterior radiograph of the pelvis showed severe ankylosis of the right hip.

Phase 1: Motor Diagnosis

(a) Identification of motor alteration:
   - Do you (or the patient in your care) have any discomfort or difficulty of any origin, when making any movement with any part of your body and/or when moving from one place to another? YES
   - Do you (or the patient in your care) have any inability, of any origin, to make any movement with any part of your body and/or to move from one place to another? YES

(b) Triaxial method of diagnosis of Dysmobility:

Axis 1. Form of presentation:

- Did these mobility problems start slowly or rather abruptly? Abruptly.

Axis 2. Evolution time:

- How long have you/the patient in your care had mobility problems? 3 years

Axis 3: D-STAGING

- **First question**: identification of the usual motor segment.
- On average, during the past month, does the patient spend most of the day standing, sitting, or lying down? Standing

Next: If the patient spends most of the day standing:

- Do you remain standing without help? Yes: Dysmobility 1-A

The Dysmobility map for clinical case 2 can be reviewed in Table 8.3.

The patient was referred to traumatology, where it was decided to evaluate surgical management. The bone scan was negative for active infection, so it was decided to perform total arthroplasty.

Bone densitometry resulted in varied osteopenia, starting management with denosumab and supplementation with calcium + vitamin D due to low plasma levels of the latter.

This case alerts us to three situations of interest:

1. Functionality may be well preserved in demobilised patients, masking significant suffering for a long time: Functionality and mobility ***are not the same things***.
2. It is possible, in some cases, to return patients to normal: After 2 weeks of rehabilitation, the patient had regained stable autonomous walking without technical aids and could sit and stand up on her own without pain. He returned to driving after a month of treatment.
3. There are conditions, such as osteopenia in this case, that must be studied and treated, to avoid, as far as possible, that the remedy of the present could become the complication of the future.

Table 8.3 Dysmobility map clinical case 2 (acute old Dysmobility)

Level	Diagnostic	Management
Motor	**Form of presentation** Acute Dysmobility	**Level of care**: Ambulatory—in-hospital
	Time of evolution Old Dysmobility	**Priority in care**: Outpatient referral for probable surgical management. It is not urgent, but it must be done quickly to avoid further loss of functionality and the occurrence of complications **Health team**: Geriatrician, radiologist, orthopaedic surgeons, rehabilitators
	D-STAGING stage Stage 1 **D-STAGING substages**: Substage A	**Level of care**: Ambulatory → hospitalised → ambulatory **General objectives**: Avoid progression Return to the best previous stage

(continued)

Table 8.3 (continued)

Level	Diagnostic	Management
Diseases	**Basal conditions**	**Define main aetiology of Dysmobility**: Severe left coxarthrosis secondary to septic arthritis **Objectives**: Rule out osteomyelitis or active septic arthritis Perform total arthroplasty
	Complications	**Existing**: search, study, and treat – Left adductor tendinitis **Risk**: Prevent – Falls, fractures, osteoporosis
Social	**Existing**	**Describe**: Wife and co-workers 2 sons abroad, the patient does not want to involve them in care **Include**: Written material is generated explaining the patient's condition, to be read by co-workers The care of the total prosthesis is explained to the patient and wife **Train**: Delivery of graphic material on underlying diseases **Stabilise**: Emotional support and health help Definition of therapeutic objectives

Case 3: Slow Old Dysmobility

Woman, 75 years old, her own house activities. She lives in a rural area, and she is supported by the family of each of her three sons and three daughters, who lived very close around on the same rural property. The patient and her family are actively involved in community life. The patient's sons and daughters are worried because they have observed that the patient is spending a lot of time sitting; it is difficult for her to get up and she no longer participates as many in visits to family members.

When consulted, the patient reports total self-worth in the basic activities of daily living (Barthel 100) but that her knees hurt a lot. The pain is very strong at the beginning of the day, but it decreases later with physical activity. However, at night, there are times when, when moving while she sleeps, she wakes up from the pain.

After lunch, she sits down and then has a hard time starting the walk again due to her pain. She also states that, although she can do it, due to the pain in her knees, she has a hard time getting up from the couch.

She walks in her house without major difficulties, and she does not use canes, but she does lean on the furniture in the house and on the walls because she feels very 'unstable'. However, when she goes out to the yard or she goes to visit her children and grandchildren, she uses a wooden cane, reaching her houses with great difficulty and having to sit all afternoon.

Finally, she says that sitting for so long bores her and makes her very anxious, so she has begun to eat more and gain weight and that she is sleeping poorly.

The physical examination revealed a height of 1.61 m, weight of 88 kilos, generalised sarcopenia, increased volume of both knees, and hard, not painful, on palpation, with a range of flexion of 25° bilaterally, without specific pain on palpation of the enthesis and tendons.

She brings frontal and lateral knee X-rays from 5 years ago, normal. The radiological study of the pelvis at the time of consultation showed severe bilateral osteoarthritis of the hips.

Phase 1: Motor Diagnosis

(a) Identification of motor alteration:

- Do you (or the patient in your care) have any discomfort or difficulty of any origin, when making any movement with any part of your body and/or when moving from one place to another? **YES**
- Do you (or the patient in your care) have any inability, of any origin, to make any movement with any part of your body and/or to move from one place to another? **YES**

(b) Triaxial method of diagnosis of Dysmobility

Axis 1. Form of presentation:

- Did these mobility problems start slowly or rather abruptly? **Slowly**.

Axis 2. Evolution time:

- How long have you/the patient in your care had mobility problems? **5 years**

Axis 3: D-STAGING
First question: identification of the usual motor segment

- On average, during the last month, did the patient spend most of the day standing, sitting, or lying down? **Sitting**

Next: If the patient spends most of the day sitting:

- Can you sit and/or stand up alone, without help? **Yes**: **Dysmobility 2-A**

The Dysmobility map for clinical case 3 can be reviewed in Table 8.4.

The Yesavage Test was applied, obtaining 5 points. No pharmacological management was initiated to evaluate the impact of the rehabilitation intervention on mood.

D'Aubigne-Postel test of 9 points (pain 3, mobility 2, gait 5 = bad).

Laboratory tests were requested [CBC, insulin curve, lipid profile, cyanocobalaminemia, albuminemia, thyroid profile, vitamin D3], which were normal.

Obesity management began with diet therapy, managed with a nutritionist, with the aim of regularizing intake and reducing weight, reaching 75 kilos in 6 months, with a notable decrease in painful symptoms.

Table 8.4 Dysmobility map clinical case 3 (slow old Dysmobility)

Level	Diagnosis	Management
Motor	**Form of presentation**: Slow Dysmobility	**Level of care**: Ambulatory—hospitalised
	Time of evolution: Old Dysmobility	**Priority in care**: Outpatient referral for probable surgical management. It is not urgent, but it must be done soon to avoid further loss of functionality and the occurrence of complications **Team**: Geriatrician, orthopaedic surgeon, physiotherapists
	D-STAGING: Stage 2 **D-STAGING SUBSTAGES**: Substage A	**Level of care** Ambulatory—hospitalised—ambulatory/community **General objectives** Avoid progression Return to the best previous stage
Diseases	**Basal conditions**	**Define main aetiology of Dysmobility**: Severe primary coxarthrosis Obesity **Objectives**: Lose weight Perform total arthroplasty
	Complications	**Existing**: Search, study, management of – Depression **Risk**: Prevent – Falls, fractures, osteoporosis
Social	**Existing**	**Describe**: Husband, three daughters, and three sons with their respective families, all implicated as caregivers **Include** Written material is generated explaining the patient's condition, to be read by co-workers The importance of maintaining adequate weight and functionality is explained to the husband. The care of the total prosthesis is explained in writing **Train** Delivery of graphic material on underlying diseases **Stabilise** Definition of therapeutic objectives

Kinesiological management to strengthen axial muscles and pelvic girdle, gait, and balance.

Mood was reevaluated after 8 months in consultation, with Yesavage = 0. However, the D'Aubigne-Postel test showed only optimization of pain, maintaining mediocre motor and walking performance, with a discrete improvement at 12 points (pain 4, mobility 2, gait 5).

Due to a good functional prognosis and good but incomplete initial response, she was referred to traumatology, performing total arthroplasty of the right hip first and, after 2 months, of the left hip, with good evolution.

In parallel, nursing carried out a home visit, detecting risk points and generating an implementation guide for environmental improvements of railings, lighting, paved roads, and elimination of obstacles.

One year after the consultation, the patient was in a state of self-sufficiency, with good care of her prosthesis, without reporting falls or complications, without weight gain, with good quality of sleep, and having resumed her usual level of activity.

Special Clinical Cases

With the following cases, we want to emphasise:

(a) The diagnostic method of Dysmobility facilitates interdisciplinarity, by allowing health professionals, not only physicians, to be able, from their own area of experience, to propose chains of causality and specific approaches. This facilitates the creation of interdisciplinary maps of causality and treatment, optimizing the interaction of health teams and the general management of the patient and her social environment.
(b) It is perfectly possible for the Dysmobility diagnostic process to be carried out by non-medical professionals, with training in geriatrics. We recommend that it is essential to complement the process with an interdisciplinary vision.
(c) By being based on concepts of quality, with a longitudinal view on the time axis, the Dysmobility diagnostic method

allows identifying the potential effects of conditions that could be considered 'banal' or of little importance. Thus, these can be included and managed, avoiding a merely transversal approach.

(d) The diagnostic method of Dysmobility allows us to propose chains of causality. This allows us to visualise more clearly not only the aetiologies but also the processes that are altered, facilitating the generation and implementation of highly consistent and comprehensive management plans.

(e) It is very possible that, after applying the method, and obtaining a map of causality chains, the initial diagnostic panorama made with the traditional method changes quite radically.

Special Clinical Case 1: Dysmobility in Geriatric Dentistry

Male, 72 years old, independent (Barthel 100), owner of a fleet of taxis, works supervising its operation. He lives with his wife and daughter. Background: active smoking, 2 cigarettes a day for >40 years, non-insulin requiring DM2, treated with metformin. He attended a geriatric consultation due to repeated torticollis. The current episode, on the right, began 2 days ago, with no relief after general measures and NAIDS. The previous one had been 1 month ago, on the same side, and 3 months ago I had had another one, but on the left side.

The spouse explains that the episodes began approximately 3 years ago, the first time she was treated with cyclobenzaprine, but the medication, although it was effective for the pain, caused agitation compatible with active delirium, so he did not use it again. Since then, he has suffered from torticollis once or twice a year, and his primary care physician would have told him that this was 'normal'. Each time the episode occurred, he was prescribed bed rest for 3 days, with oral and topical anti-inflammatories. To sleep and relax the muscles, Pregabalin 75 mg every 8 h was indicated. At the time of the consultation, he had already had 4 episodes in 6 months, so he decided to see a specialist.

The patient's spouse adds that the patient moves a lot at night, snores, and makes a noise like he is 'rubbing a finger on wet glass'.

The physical examination revealed a respiratory rate of 24/min and painful contracture of the right sternocleidomastoid with an antalgic posture of the neck and head. Significant halitosis. Teeth in poor condition, tooth attrition, and multiple caries lesions.

Blood tests were requested including vitamin B12 levels (because of the use of metformin), antero-posterior chest X-ray, and spirometry; and geriatric dentistry was consulted with a diagnosis of dental caries and possible bruxism/grinding. General education about oral hygiene was carried out.

Phase 1. Motor Diagnosis

(a) Identification of motor alteration:

- Do you (or the patient in your care) have any discomfort or difficulty of any origin, when making any movement with any part of your body and/or when moving from one place to another? YES
- Do you (or the patient in your care) have any inability, of any origin, to make any movement with any part of your body and/or to move from one place to another? YES

(b) Triaxial method of diagnosis of Dysmobility

Axis 1. Form of presentation:

- Did these mobility problems start slowly or rather abruptly? Fast, abruptly.

Axis 2. Evolution time:

- How long have you/the patient in your care had mobility problems? 3 years

Axis 3: D-STAGING

First question: identification of the usual motor segment.

- On average, during the last month, did the patient spend most of the day standing, sitting, or lying down? Standing

Next: If the patient spends most of the day standing:

- Do you walk without help? Yes: Dysmobility 1-A

The Dysmobility map for special clinical case 1 can be reviewed in Table 8.5.

Plasma vitamin B12 levels were low (93 pg/mL). Chest X-ray showed costal horizontalization with moderate bilateral hyperinflation and ruled out nodular images. Spirometry was compatible with a moderate chronic obstructive pattern, diagnosing chronic obstructive pulmonary disease.

Treatment was started with oral vitamin B complex for 30 days and then intramuscular maintenance every 4 months, anticholinergic/LABA (umeclidinium 55/vilanterol 22) 1 daily dose. According to the patient and his family, treatment with bupropion was started to support smoking cessation.

Geriatric dentistry confirmed the presence of dental caries at the level of premolars and bruxism while awake and sleeping. He implemented the extraction of two teeth and subsequent rehabilitation with implants. Finally, occlusion management with a relaxation plane.

Pregabalin 75 mg was maintained in very low doses (1/2 per night) for 3 months.

After a year, the patient had not presented torticollis again; he had rarely relapsed into smoking (in the context of his work). No halitosis, with good oral hygiene. He had no respiratory complications, with a respiratory rate of 18/min. The sleeping pattern had normalised; he no longer moved during the night, and the noises had disappeared. He and his family had resumed the practice of going out on weekend excursions, something he had stopped doing years ago due to easy fatigue.

Table 8.5 Dysmobility map special clinical case 1 (geriatric dentistry)

Level	Diagnosis	Management
Motor	**Form of presentation** Acute Dysmobility	Level of care: Ambulatory
	Time of evolution Old Dysmobility	Health attention priority: Not urgent, requires evaluation to find and treat aetiologies and complications Health team: Geriatrist, geriatric dentist
	D-STAGING stages Stage 1 **D-STAGING substages**: Substage A	Level of attention Ambulatory Set general objectives: Avoid progression Return to the best previous stage
Diseases	**Basal conditions**	Define the main aetiology of Dysmobility: Vigilance and sleep bruxism Smoking Investigate probable causes
	Complications	Existing: Research, study, and treat – Dental caries – Chronic obstructive pulmonary disease Absent: Prevent – Vitamin B12 deficiency secondary to metformin use – Osteoporosis, lung cancer
Social	**Existing**	Describe Wife, 1 daughter, implicated in the care. Both nonsmoking Including Written material is generated that explains the importance of maintaining oral hygiene, quitting smoking, and annual control by geriatric dentistry Train Delivery of graphic material on underlying diseases Stabilise Definition of therapeutic objectives

Special Clinical Case 2: Dysmobility in Logopedics

Woman, 65 years old, previously totally self-sufficient, lived alone, began to have frequent forgetfulness after 1 year of evolution. Evaluated by neurology, a major neurocognitive disorder of a mixed degenerative-vascular neurocognitive disorder was diagnosed. In an initial phase, treatment with memantine began, and it was suggested to prevent the patient from living alone, so she went to live with her son and his family (her son, his wife, and their two daughters).

After 3 months, she evolved with progressive loss of interest in her environment and loss of appetite. The family observed that she spent most of the day sitting, almost without moving, and they took her to geriatrics, where an important decrease in verbal communication, paleness, and weight loss was observed. Depressive disorder was diagnosed, in the context of iron-deficient anaemia, vitamins D and B12 deficiency, and sarcopenia. Corresponding treatments begin. Due to difficulties in communication between the patient and the family, management is suggested by logopedics.

Phase 1: Motor Diagnosis

(a) Motor alteration identification:
  - Do you (or the patient in charge) have any discomfort or difficulty of any origin, when performing some movement with any part of your body and/or when moving from one place to another? YES
  - Do you (or the patient in charge) have any impossibility, of any origin, to perform some movement with any part of your body and/or to move from one place to another? YES

(b) Triaxial Dysmobility Method

Axis 1. Form of presentation:

- Did these mobility problems start slowly or rather abruptly? Fast.

Axis 2. Evolution time:

- How long have you/the patient in your care had mobility problems? 3 months

Axis 3: D-STAGING
First question: identification of the usual motor segment.

- On average, during the last month, did the patient spend most of the day standing, sitting, or lying down? Sitting

Following:
If the patient spends most of the day sitting:

- Do you sit and get up without help? Yes: Dysmobility 2-A

The Dysmobility map for special clinical case 2 can be reviewed in Table 8.6.

Table 8.6 Dysmobility map special clinical case 2 (logopedics)

Level	Diagnostic	Management
Motor	**Form of presentation** Acute Dysmobility	**Level of health care**: Ambulatory
	Time of evolution Recent Dysmobility	**Health attention priority**: Not urgent, requires evaluation to find and treat aetiologies and complications **Health team**: Geriatrist, logopedist
	D-STAGING phases Stage 2 **D-STAGING subphases**: Substage A	**Level of attention**: Ambulatory **Set general objectives**: Avoid progression Return to the best previous stage

(continued)

Table 8.6 (continued)

Level	Diagnostic	Management
Diseases	**Basal conditions**	**Define the main aetiology of Dysmobility**: Dysphagia, gastroesophageal reflux, sleep disorder **Objective**: Define probable causes
	Complications	**Existing**: **Research, study, and treat** – *Helicobacter pylori* pangastritis – Anaemia – Deficiency of iron, vitamins D and B12 – Sarcopenia – Depression **Absent**: Prevent – Progression of major neurocognitive disease – Falls
Social	**Existing**	**Describe**: A son and his wife, both implicated in care **Including**: Written material is generated that explains the importance of maintaining oral hygiene, quitting smoking, and annual control by geriatric dentistry **Train**: Delivery of graphic material on underlying diseases **Stabilise**: Definition of therapeutic objectives

After the logopedic evaluation, mild oropharyngeal dysphagia was diagnosed, associated with odynophagia, in the context of pharyngitis. The existence of gastroesophageal reflux was raised. Derived again to geriatrics, the diagnostic entity of gastroesophageal reflux—chronic sleep disorder—was proposed.

The study (pH measurement and polysomnogram) demonstrated nocturnal gastroesophageal reflux and loss of normal sleep architecture with multiple micro-awakening.

High digestive endoscopy was diagnostic for atrophic chronic pangastritis, discarding esophagitis. The urease test for *Helicobacter pylori* was positive.

Food and sleep hygiene measures were established; along with helicobacter eradication tritherapy, nocturnal levosulpiride was added in low doses.

In the control after 6 weeks, the patient had no signs of pharyngitis or dysphagia, she had recovered her appetite, and her communication with the family was very good. It maintained a practically normal level of daily activities, including outings to make purchases, and the forgetfulness had disappeared. The mood was normal. Antidepressant management was suspended. Memantine remained; the patient stopped taking it after 6 months.

Final Comments After Solved Clinical Cases

The diagnostic method of Dysmobility facilitates interdisciplinarity, by allowing health professionals, not only doctors, to be able, from their experience and expertise, to propose chains of causality and specific approaches. This facilitates the creation of interdisciplinary maps of causality and treatment (like the Dysmobility map), optimizing the interaction of health teams and the general management of the patient and the social environment.

It is perfectly possible for the Dysmobility diagnostic process to be carried out by non-medical professionals, with training in geriatrics. In any case, it is essential to complement the process with an interdisciplinary vision, including a trained physician.

By being based on concepts of quality, with a longitudinal view on the time axis, the Dysmobility diagnostic method allows identifying the potential effects of conditions that could be considered 'banal' or of little importance. Thus, these can be included and managed, avoiding a merely cross-sectional approach.

The diagnostic method of Dysmobility allows us to propose chains of causality. This allows us to visualise more clearly not only the aetiologies but also the processes that are altered, facilitating the generation and implementation of highly consistent and comprehensive management plans.

It is very possible that, after applying the method and obtaining a map of causality chains, the initial diagnostic panorama made with the traditional method changes quite radically.

9 Dysmobility and Aging: From Clinical Dysmobility to the Movement-Time Theory

Introduction

In Chap. 1, we proposed a clinical definition of movement (continuous phenomenon, composed of the constant spatiotemporal changes made by a body and/or occurring in a body and/or received by a body).

We then proposed that what matters to us in the clinical setting are the effects that movement generates on biological systems.

Finally, we proposed a definition of health based on movement: '***state of perfect mobility***'. This means that, in a state of perfect health, all systems, all components, are in perfect motor balance. On the other hand, health would be affected when altered or deleterious movements appear or necessary movements disappear.

In this chapter, we will briefly lay the foundations of the Movement-Time Theory, a theory that seeks to unify the understanding of a universal phenomenon: aging. Depending on the point of view, we could also call this the Dysmobility Theory.

From Perfection to Imperfection

We could relativise the concept of 'perfection' and say that health is a state of mobility in which we can thrive as individuals or 'feel' good. However, this would actually mean relativizing our

J. L. Dinamarca-Montecinos, *Dysmobility in Geriatrics*,
https://doi.org/10.1007/978-3-031-72716-0_9

definition of health, since we know that we can thrive as individuals even in significant states of illness and that the 'feeling' of well-being does not exclude the presence of serious illnesses. So, we will insist on how important the 'perfection' of mobility is, and we will emphasise other aspects that will allow us to understand that the definition is applicable and practical.

The movements a person can experience are not always evident to them. Indeed, the most impressive movements occur at the macro and micro scales that make them imperceptible at first glance. Good examples of this are the movements of the Earth, including rotation (the turning of the planet on its own axis). Rotation is responsible for the days and nights we experience continually. We do not perceive the Earth's rotation, which occurs at a speed of approximately 1670 km/h, but we do perceive the day-night cycle, and our body has evolved for millions of years, preferring daytime activity and night-time rest, adapting the physiology of the species at both a molecular and social level, generating what is now known as the '24-h biological clock' that governs the circadian cycle.

The circadian rhythm is a motor pattern that helps our bodies keep track of time, and this is necessary to maintain homeostasis and the health of living organisms. While pivotal to health, these processes are 'silent' to us on a day-to-day basis, and we are not always aware of them. Indeed, most cells in the body have molecular clocks interconnected by transcription/translation feedback loops [1].

An interesting exception is the pluripotent stem cells (a type of stem cell abundant during the development of the embryo and that subsists in some nuclei or 'niches' related to some specific tissues during adult stages), which lack circadian oscillations, and we consider them 'uncoupled from time'. We don't understand this very well yet, but it is being considered that the central circadian clock mechanism is negatively regulated in them, both at the genetic and epigenetic levels and in the interaction with other clocks in the circadian clock network which regulate homeostasis. It is possible that the circadian clock significantly influences the generation of pluripotency and cellular reprogramming [1].

This literature on circadian rhythms and the biological clock has taught us that, to regenerate certain parts of our body, we need cells capable of being 'available 24/7'. For this availability to be effective, these cells cannot be 'awake' or 'asleep' but rather 'dormant' or 'standing by' outside the influence of the 24-h biological clock, and they remain this way throughout our lives, until differentiation is necessary. However, once the stem cells come out of their stand-by state, since they have received the order to collaborate in the repair of a serious tissue problem, they 'enter in the time dimension', which condemns them to its laws, including maturation and deterioration. These cells thus belong to a kind of 'Asimovian universe' (in the sense of Isaac Asimov's novel *The End of Eternity* [2]. However, to be frank, this does not mean that stem cells do not age.

Returning to our movements that are difficult to perceive, they (terrestrial rotation, circadian rhythm, and sleep-wake cycle) are certainly of enormous importance for our lives, but we are not always aware of them. Any modification of its patterns generates important effects on our lives and, certainly, on our health. Although the Earth's rotation has not changed significantly in the last several thousand years, we have changed our volitional response (our 'lifestyles') to the circadian cycle. In fact, we take away hours from our night's rest and, because of various conditions and diseases (obesity, depression, vitamin deficiencies), we suffer serious health problems during sleep (insomnia, sleep apnoea), which prevent us from resting properly.

In a 2018 study in Mexico, 18.8% of the population suffered from insomnia and 27.3% of the adult population suffered from obstructive sleep apnoea [3]. Various Mendelian randomisation studies causally associate sleep disorders with serious entities such as dementia, stroke, myocardial infarction, cerebrovascular accidents, cancer, rheumatoid arthritis, obesity, and hyperuricemia [4–6].

Despite the striking prevalence of sleep disorders and their association with wider pathology, proportionally little is known about the connection between sleep deprivation and problems of motor aetiology [7]. Sleep disorders have never been considered 'problems of motor aetiology' (we prefer to consider them the origin of other problems). To be honest, human beings are also not very actively willing to change those motor patterns called 'life-styles' that underlie these and other disorders. However, it is undeniable that the interrelation between the Earth's cycles and our own biological cycles has a level of immutability and perfection, which we take care of spoiling day by day. Is it possible to achieve motor perfection?

Is There a Relationship Between Movement, Its Disorders, and Aging?

We have seen that movement patterns and health are related, and not just related but closely related. So, it is okay to ask the question that titles this section. Since both movement and aging are inherent and unavoidable processes of the life cycle, how are they related to each other?

Topics related to aging have been an important stimulus for the development of science since ancient times. Among others, the quest for 'eternal youth' by medieval alchemists led to the first experiments and defined the rudiments of modern science. In parallel with the phenomenon of epidemiological transition and population aging, since the end of the Second World War, various theories have been defined that seek to explain aging from different perspectives [8, 9].

Biological theories of aging seek to understand the aging of living organisms from two fundamental points of view, which classify them in turn into stochastic (random or external) and non-stochastic (cellular, programming, or internal) theories. Both groups support a set of various lines of thought and experimentation. Below, we briefly describe them.

– Stochastic theories [10]:

  The paradigm of stochastic theories is the Theory of Free Radicals, proposed by Denham Harman in 1956 and updated several times by its author.

Conceptually, these theories look for the causes of aging in the 'environment', whether external, surrounding the cells, or intracellular (especially peri-mitochondrial).

They define aging as the accumulation of changes that generate an increased risk of death.

- Non-stochastic theories [11, 12]:

  Its paradigm is the Biological Clock Theory, proposed by Leonard Hayflick in 1961.

  They seek to explain aging through the execution of programs by biological control systems, fundamentally intracellular.

  They define aging as the sum of the aging of cells, programmed with a specific limit for each cell line, which determines that, when the time comes, the cell can no longer divide.

Although interesting advances have been made in understanding the deterioration of living systems, in optimizing the number of years they live (longevity); in the prevention, approach, and treatment of diseases in older people (geriatrics); and in the ways to achieve the best functionality and independence (gerontology), fundamental questions remain that we have not yet resolved.

Now, we propose some answers to these questions, based on the analysis of the Movement-Time Theory, which I proposed for the first time in 2006 [13] and which is based on a new definition of aging.

Movement-Time Theory or Dysmobility Theory

It is based on the following four foundations:

1. We find ourselves inhabiting a space-time universe.
2. Everything that exists in this space-time universe moves.
3. Everything that exists in this space-time universe ages.
4. Time, movement, and aging are interdependent.

Based on these foundations, aging is defined as:

The product of the interaction between movement and time.

From this definition, seven main characteristics of aging emerge, which are presented below:

1. Aging is a constant process that occurs in all elements, living and non-living (including ideas, philosophies, cultures, etc.).
2. Aging generates, in parallel, two effects: deterioration and maturation. There is no aging that is only deteriorative or only maturative. We live in a dynamic balance between both. In this way, 'deteriorating' aging is that which occurs due to 'deleterious', 'absent', and/or 'altered' movements, and 'healthy' (or "maturative") aging is that which is achieved through 'protective' movements. Therefore, AGING DOES NOT ONLY GENERATE DETERIORATION.
3. Aging is an inter- and transgenerational continuum: It does not begin or end; it just continues. In other words, we have begun to age before we were conceived, and our current aging is part of the aging of our offspring.
4. Aging is an original continuum: We all age in different ways.
5. Aging is an interpersonal continuum: The aging of one person influences the way others age. That is, we all age in complementary ways.
6. Aging is a multidimensional continuum: biopsychosocial and spiritual, functional, cultural, architectural, artistic, etc.
7. Aging is a reversible continuum. We can influence some elements to limit or reverse deterioration or enhance maturation, producing healthy aging. Unfortunately, the opposite is also possible.

Below, we analyse these points based on some questions that we have all asked ourselves at some point in our lives.

What Is Aging?

Aging generates, in parallel, two effects: deterioration and maturation.

As a general rule, we consider aging as a process of deterioration. Also, as we move through time, the signs of this deterioration become increasingly evident. However, it is no less true that, as we move through time, we also develop skills, create links, and carry out undertakings and achievements, generating knowledge and wisdom. All this, clearly, is not a sign of deterioration.

As obvious as it may seem, these things also happen 'over the years', that is, they are not achieved from one moment to the next. Aged wine and cheese have more value, more 'body', colour, tone, and flavour. If we dedicate ourselves to exclusively studying the deteriorating effects of aging, we will be missing a large part of the process.

On the other hand, it is convenient to consider that, although aging does indeed lead to deterioration, this is heterogeneous. Depending on various genetic and environmental factors, people reach different levels of deterioration, regardless of the chronological years lived. In other words, two people of the same age can have very different levels of impairment and, of course, very different levels of development (or 'maturation') as well.

In this way, it becomes clear that it is not only the chronologically accumulated time that influences aging but also the different ways in which our organisms behave during these chronological units of time. Those behaviours can be measured in terms of movement. There are different types of movement at different structural levels: molecular movement, genetic movement, and movement of tissues, organs, and systems, which develop over time seeking the greatest possible maturation with the least possible wear. If the movements are deteriorating, in the same unit of chronological time, there will be more deterioration than if the movements are protective or 'maturative'.

Thus, the accumulated chronological time (which we commonly call 'age') ceases to be a 'risk factor' but rather becomes a way of objectifying the amount of deterioration associated with various types of behaviour, that is, to different movement patterns. This constitutes a good explanation for the fact that there are centenarian people who have excellent levels of health and very young people who have serious deterioration: It seems more appropriate to consider aging a process of parallel wear and maturation, rather than just a process of wear or deterioration.

When Do We Start to Age?

Aging neither begins nor ends: It just continues.

This question may not have an exact answer from a chronological point of view. One does not begin to age at a certain point in space-time, but rather one continues to age. The originality of each individual is developing long before the gametes that make it come together. The genetic materials of each of these gametes have been encoding a history—a 'genetic history'—that can literally go back to the very beginning of time [14–16].

Seen this way, living beings begin to age 'before' existing and continue to age 'after' dying. Biological life is a continuum of specific (and sometimes interspecific) transfer of encoded genetic information. The experiences transmitted 'from generation to generation' acquire an unsuspected value: They are not only transmitted while individuals from different generations interact in a way—let's call it that—'in person', but they have already been transmitted in a complementary way through the genetic material which, looked at this way, is especially suitable for learning, perfecting, and retransmitting these experiences. The death of an individual, or of a generation of individuals, does not put an end to their own aging, which will be perpetuated in subsequent generations. Yes, we could say that a species stops aging when it becomes completely extinct.

A good example of this is that, through the study of mitochondrial DNA through the maternal line, we can go back to the very origins of the human species. Aging neither begins nor ends: It just continues.

How Do We Age?

Aging is an inter- and transgenerational continuum, original, interpersonal, multidimensional, and reversible.

We can respond from two perspectives: understanding aging as a process of living species and understanding it as a phenomenon in itself.

In the first case, we must say that, although a cross-sectional look at the chronological axis is completely valid, it will only give us limited information about aging in the 'present' of a species: of a few generations or of a single individual.

Aging is a generational issue: We do not age individually but rather generationally—more precisely, trans-generationally. In reality, aging is individual only in the sense that generations are made up of individuals.

Therefore, if we want to look at aging from a chronological point of view, we must do so more broadly: Aging has a past, a present, and a future that go far beyond the past, present, and future of a single person or generation.

On the other hand, describing how we age from a phenomenological point of view can be a little more complex: It depends on a set of functions between [6] movement and time. Our results have suggested that the determinants of this function are varied and simultaneous, depending on the structural level that they directly affect.

According to this, they can be, for example, simple (the movement of one type of enzyme correcting neuronal DNA replication) or integrated (the coordinated movement of all corrective systems for neuronal DNA replication), molecular (a part of a domain of a type of enzyme), or systemic (the peristaltic coordination of the digestive system).

The type of aging that each level has will depend on how its components move: how coordinated they are, how their regulatory systems work, how efficient they are in removing toxic substances, the speed at which they manage to cover the needs of other systems, etc.

Thus, we can say that living organisms carry out movements that allow them to fulfil functions, allowing survival. Along with that, as something inherent to the relationship between movement and time, movement generates a deterioration (e.g. oxidative) and, at the same time, an improvement of the systems. The best movements will be repeated and perfected and passed on to the next generation, both through genetic information and through imitation learning and cultural and social conditioning. Therefore, constantly, continuously, and in parallel, we are subjected to various levels of deterioration and improvement.

Final Thoughts on Movement-Time: Why Do We Age?

This question is tricky because, when we have asked it, it is generally to try to explain the reasons for the DETERIORATION. Nobody asks much about why we manage to evolve, be better, and get what we want and need. The ultimate goal of movement is our well-being, so if our movements generated well-being for us, it was what we wanted and expected, and that's all.

If we consider our definition of aging, we could say that we age because we move in time. Paraphrasing Descartes, we can say that '*I move, therefore, I am*'.

Modifying aging, then, depends on whether we can modify time and/or movement.

Modifying Time

Someday, we will, perhaps, be able to manipulate time. (And, when we die, we will certainly leave time.) For now, the best option is to optimise our movements. That is, move better in time.

As we saw previously, it seems that stem cells 'go out' of time. In them, deterioration and maturation are limited or conditioned, since they are in a state of latency or 'stand-by', which we still do not fully understand. What we do know is that a large amount of energy is invested in maintaining a favourable environment around these cells, the so-called 'nests' or 'niches' of stem cells.

However, stem cells do age [17], and, together with alterations in their niches, many of their causes of aging depend on intrinsic pathways, their own. So, in effect, there are both intrinsic (cellular or programmed) and extrinsic (random) causes. These causes become more frequent as the time that the cells have been alive increases, that is, they are more frequent in older individuals [18, 19].

So, this apparent 'magic of leaving time' of stem cells is not real. It is not possible (at least for now) to exit time without dying. Time surrounds us and permeates us, so if we wanted to exempt ourselves from deterioration (the way stem cells do), we would at the same time have to renounce maturation, along with putting a huge amount of resources at the service of that. It is a way of 'being' without 'existing'.

In reality, temporal latency systems are not forms of time manipulation but rather ways of tricking our body into maintaining it without suffering the most abrupt and deleterious effects of the interaction between movement and time, that is, moving without deteriorating too much but without maturing either. Basically, they are equivalent to the use of different movements so that a biological body 'stagnates' in a temporal latency. Indeed, this would be achieved by applying a set of movements, that is, generating work and expending energy, not by the organism itself but by an external system, which could be a machine. This is possible, although still in the experimental phase [1] and, at the cellular level, not at the level of an entire organism.

The benefits of an achievement of this magnitude are clear: We would delay the deterioration associated with aging, we would be able to travel great distances such as interstellar distances, and we would increase our longevity. However, we would continue to age, as soon as we left the 'nest' that was transforming us into 'stem cells', and, even then, the intrinsic mechanisms of deterioration would appear sooner or later.

For now, as our understanding of stem cell aging advances, it seems very likely to optimise the deterioration associated with aging, by optimizing or reversing the deterioration of deleterious conditions that affect stem cells [20].

Modifying Movement

Why do we age, then? Because we move in time. In the temporal dimension, movement, generated to achieve benefits, not only generates benefits but also deteriorations, depending largely on how we perform our movements. Apparently, no matter how well we move, over time there will always be a 'remaining deterioration', inherent to the use of energy and the generation of cumulative damage, oxidative stress, and repair failures.

What we must remember is that we can optimise aging and make it 'healthy' or 'successful', generating changes in our movements that have beneficial impacts by reducing deterioration and its mechanisms or by reducing its impact on the generation of cascades of deterioration.

What Is the Interaction Between Movement and Time?

In 2007, I tried to answer this question based on an experiment [21]. Two groups of people in the bedridden phase and with a diagnosis of depression were subjected to two different measures. In the first group, a new concept was applied, which we called 'minimum necessary movement', defined as:

Minimum Necessary Movement (MNM)
Minimum set of motor actions and their frequency of execution, necessary to produce a deleterious or protective effect on a significant percentage of the sample to which it is applied.

In this case, the minimum necessary movement consisted of a physical change in the patient's usual position, from bed to chair, for 1 h a day. In the second group, translational movement was not applied but cognitive movement, a conversation for 1 h a day.

Both groups were maintained for a month in this dynamic, after which the scores on the Yesavage scale [22] changed significantly in the first group, improving, while in the second group, they remained the same.

This meant that the minimum necessary movement applied in group 1 (a movement of position changes in spacetime) was sufficient to improve their health indicators and aging prognosis, while the minimum necessary cognitive movement was insufficient to achieve this effect in group 2.

On the other hand, the more time passed, the greater the impact of the minimum necessary movement on Yesavage values.

Although many experiences and data are lacking, in this sample, it was possible to see that a specific movement was capable of reversing the negative effects of a disease on aging, producing healthy aging. In the same way, a repetitive movement can cause damage, as in the case of some occupational and sports diseases.

This apparently simple experience allowed us to postulate that the function between movement and time occurs in the form of a product. Aging would be the product of the interaction between movement and time:

$$\boldsymbol{E = M^{*}t}$$

where '*E*' is aging, '*M*' is movement, and '*t*' is time.

If we talk about literal definitions, the following is the new definition of aging proposed by the Time-Movement Theory:

Aging: Product of the interaction between movement and time.

We can call this theory Movement Time Theory. We can also call it Dysmobility Theory or, depending on the point of view, *Eumobility* Theory (from the ancient Greek 'eu' (substantive): correct, perfect).

The equation may require many adjustments, for example, to include the importance of 'space', a modifiable variable closely related to time—also, to express the nuances related to protection systems and the differences between maturative and deteriorating aging.

However, as it stands, it allows us to understand aging from a comprehensive and integrative perspective, emphasizing how fundamental movement is in our lives.

Final Comments

The aging process is still a topic of research and reflection. The Movement-Time Theory allows access to a broader vision of it, limiting the pejorative conception linked to the concept of 'aging'. It allows a more specific look at the concept of aging itself, rather than its causes or effects. By considering aging a function between movement and time, it opens new and important perspectives for intervention. By considering it a continuous and trans-generational process, it involves with the development of the human species itself. Finally, by depending largely on the interaction of different types of movement, it allows access to various levels of reversibility of deterioration. To age better we cannot (yet) modify time, but we can modify the way we move.

References

1. Agriesti F, Cela O, Capitanio N. "Time is out of joint" in pluripotent stem cells: how and why. Int J Mol Sci. 2024;25(4):2063. https://doi.org/10.3390/ijms25042063.
2. Asimov I. The end of eternity. 1st ed. New York: Doubleday Science Fiction; 1955.
3. Guerrero-Zúñiga S, Gaona-Pineda EB, Cuevas-Nasu L, Torre-Bouscoulet L, Reyes-Zúñiga M, Shamah-Levy T, Pérez-Padilla R. Prevalencia de síntomas de sueño y riesgo de apnea obstructiva del sueño en México. Salud Publica Mex. 2018;60(3):347–55. https://doi.org/10.21149/9280.
4. Sambou ML, Zhao X, Hong T, Wang N, Dai J. Associations between sleep-behavioral traits and healthspan: a one-sample Mendelian randomization study based on 388,909 participants of the UK-biobank. J Affect Disord. 2024;350:854–62. https://doi.org/10.1016/j.jad.2024.01.122.
5. Gao RC, Sang N, Jia CZ, Zhang MY, Li BH, Wei M, Wu GC. Association between sleep traits and rheumatoid arthritis: a Mendelian randomization study. Front Public Health. 2022;10:940161. https://doi.org/10.3389/fpubh.2022.940161.
6. Lei T, Li M, Qian H, Yang J, Hu Y, Hua L. The effect of sleep on metabolism, musculoskeletal disease, and mortality in the general US population: analysis of results from the National Health and Nutrition Examination Survey. JMIR Public Health Surveill. 2023;9:e46385. https://doi.org/10.2196/46385.
7. Chun MY, Cho BJ, Yoo SH, Oh B, Kang JS, Yeon C. Association between sleep duration and musculoskeletal pain: the Korea National Health and

Nutrition Examination Survey 2010–2015. Medicine (Baltimore). 2018;97(50):e13656. https://doi.org/10.1097/MD.0000000000013656.
8. Carbajo VM. La Historia de la vejez. Ensayos. 2008;23:237–54.
9. Pérez V, Sierra F. Biología del envejecimiento. Rev Med Chile. 2009;137(2):296–302. https://doi.org/10.4067/S0034-98872009000200017.
10. Harman D. The free radical theory of aging. Antioxid Redox Signal. 2003;5(5):557–61. https://doi.org/10.1089/152308603770310202.
11. Hayflick L. Cómo y por qué envejecemos. Barcelona: Herder; 1999.
12. Diggs J. Cellular theory of aging. In: Loue SJ, Sajatovic M, editors. Encyclopedia of aging and public health. Boston: Springer; 2008. https://doi.org/10.1007/978-0-387-33754-8_81.
13. Dinamarca-Montecinos JL. Teoría del Movimiento-Tiempo: Una nueva teoría para comprender el proceso de envejecer. Bol Hosp Viña del Mar. 2015;71(4):151–3.
14. Fu Q, Posth C, Hajdinjak M, Petr M, Mallick S, Fernandes D, Furtwängler A, Haak W, et al. The genetic history of ice age Europe. Nature. 2016;534(7606):200–5. https://doi.org/10.1038/nature17993.
15. Flegontov P, Altınışık NE, Changmai P, Rohland N, Mallick S, Adamski N, Bolnick DA, Broomandkhoshbacht N, et al. Palaeo-Eskimo genetic ancestry and the peopling of Chukotka and North America. Nature. 2019;570(7760):236–40. https://doi.org/10.1038/s41586-019-1251-y.
16. Reilly PF, Tjahjadi A, Miller SL, Akey JM, Tucci S. The contribution of Neanderthal introgression to modern human traits. Curr Biol. 2022;32(18):R970–83. https://doi.org/10.1016/j.cub.2022.08.027.
17. Sharpless N, Schatten G. Stem cell aging. J Gerontol A Biol Sci Med Sci. 2009;64A(2):202–4. https://doi.org/10.1093/gerona/gln070.
18. de Haan G, Lazare S. Aging of hematopoietic stem cells. Blood. 2018;131(5):479–87.
19. Rudolph KL. Stem cell aging. Mech Ageing Dev. 2020;193:111394. https://doi.org/10.1016/j.mad.2020.111394.
20. Liu B, Qu J, Zhang W, Izpisua-Belmonte J, Liu G. A stem cell aging framework: from mechanisms to interventions. Cell Rep. 2022;41:111451. https://doi.org/10.1016/j.celrep.2022.111451.
21. Dinamarca J, Rubio R, Bonta C. Teoría de la Dismovilidad: Movimiento, tiempo y envejecimiento. In: En búsqueda de las bases de una única Teoría del Envejecimiento. Ediciones de la Fundación MAPFRE, premio Ayuda a la Investigación Ignacio de Larramendi 2007. Granada: Universidad de Granada; 2007. https://app.mapfre.com/ccm/content/documentos/fundacion/salud/becas/teoria-de-la-dismovilidad-movimientos-tiempo-y-envejecimiento.pdf.
22. Hoyl T, Valenzuela EC, Marín LPP. Depresión en el adulto mayor: evaluación preliminar de la efectividad, como instrumento de tamizaje, de la versión de 5 ítems de la Escala de Depresión Geriátrica. Rev Med Chile. 2000;128(11):1199–204. https://doi.org/10.4067/S0034-98872000001100003.

Glossary 10

Introduction

In the following glossary, we summarise the main concepts delivered in the book. They are included in five main titles: Movement, Geriatrics, Dysmobility, Aging, and Health.

Movement

- **Kinetics**: the study of everything that can influence movement [1].
- **Kinematics**: the study of movement itself [1].
- **Body**: any element that is subject to movement. This includes non-physical bodies but which are 'bodies' because they move, such as thoughts and, also, more abstract concepts such as emotions and the soul.
- **Movement (physical definition)**: change in the position of a body, over time, with respect to a reference system. The study of movement depends on physics and mechanics and, within it, kinematics and dynamics. Seen this way, movement is a phenomenon of positional dynamics that occur in time [1].
- **Movement (clinical definition)**: Continuous phenomenon, composed of the constant spatiotemporal changes made by a body/occurring in a body (or a set of bodies or all bodies).
- **Minimum necessary movement**: Minimum set of motor actions and their frequency of execution, necessary to produce

J. L. Dinamarca-Montecinos, *Dysmobility in Geriatrics*,
https://doi.org/10.1007/978-3-031-72716-0_10

a deleterious or protective effect on a significant percentage of the sample to which it is applied [2].

- **Continuous movement (concept)** [2]: Everything is in constant movement. Therefore, movement is also constantly present throughout the human economy, at all levels of the body, the mind, in the social and functional dimension and even in the spiritual one. To understand how the movement 'flows', it is good to consider various continuums such as the NEMOH [3]. NEMOH emerged evolutionary and has been perfected to facilitate our movements. Other forms of continuum are, for example, muscle chains.
- **NEMOH** [3]: Continuum of interdependent systems: neuroendocrine muscle bone haematology. It concentrates almost 100% of the calcium available in the body.

Geriatrics

- **Geriatrics (tools)** [4]:
  - **Integrality**: According to the biopsychosocial, spiritual, and functional paradigm.
  - **Interdisciplinarity**: Several disciplines working together based on agreements that, in turn, are based on the best available evidence.
  - **Various levels**: Cover all levels of care, not only outpatient and hospital but also home, community, and the interfaces between them, called 'liaison'.
  - **Staging**: Corresponds to the description of the natural history of diseases, based on the definition of key stages. These stages are turning points when it is necessary to intervene to reverse, slow, or stop the progression of a disease.
- **Geriatric syndrome (definition)** [5]: Set of signs and symptoms of diverse aetiology, highly prevalent in geriatric ages (usually over 60 years) (and/or having a minimal or much lower representation in younger ages), multifactorial, whose sustainable management requires an approach at various levels of care (preventive, acute, rehabilitation and follow-up, not only clinical but also political-organizational) and that has evidence of better results (particularly in functionality and quality

of life) with geriatric management, compared with usual or 'traditional' management.

- **Geriatric syndrome (characteristics)** [6]:
  - Self-perpetuation: Each consequence of a geriatric syndrome negatively influences others and itself. Generation of vicious circles that make recovery difficult, rather than facilitating the progression of the disease.
  - Linear progression: Or downward sloping effect. The natural history of geriatric syndromes inevitably evolves towards loss of functionality, dependency, and death if interventions are not carried out in time. Their outcomes are progressively worse. They don't 'get better on their own'.
  - Contagiousness: They have the capacity to progressively compromise social levels, from the intimacy of the family to the integrity of health systems.
  - Expansiveness: Or cluster bomb effect. One geriatric syndrome will lead to the appearance of other geriatric syndromes. Geriatric syndromes are associated with each other and attack various areas that apparently have nothing to do with each other.

Dysmobility [6, 7]

- **Dysmobility (definition)**: Geriatric syndrome, consisting of discomfort, difficulty, and/or inability to move part of the body and/or move, secondary to various pathological situations of any origin (biological, psychological, social, spiritual, functional, etc.), that affects the quality of life and/or that has a risk of progression.
- **Motor discomfort**: Mobility that allows the motor goal to be achieved, without altering the normal course of movement (motor arc) but with discomfort.
- **Motor difficulty**: Mobility that allows achieving the motor objective but altering the normal course of movement. It is not necessarily associated with discomfort.
- **Dysmobility (types)**: There are two types of Dysmobility: Acute and Slow. When combined with the time of evolution,

Acute Dysmobility can be Recent or Old, while Slow Dysmobility will always be considered Old. Both types of Dysmobility can be permanent or temporary.

- **Acute Dysmobility**: That which occurs abruptly, quickly over time.
- **Slow Dysmobility**: That which occurs slowly and progressively, sometimes almost imperceptibly.
- **Old Dysmobility**: That which, at the time of diagnosis, is more than 1 year old since the onset of signs and symptoms.
- **Recent Dysmobility**: That which, at the time of diagnosis, is less than a year old since the onset of signs and symptoms.
- **Dysmobility (moments)**: Dysmobility includes three moments which in turn determine three forms of deterioration. These are standing, sitting, and lying down. Sitting is an intermediate stage between life standing and life in bed.
- **Dysmobility (depth)**: The more advanced in time the staging level is, the more severe and 'deeper' the Dysmobility will be.
- **Dysmobility (prognosis)**: The prognosis of Dysmobility is established according to its stability. Stability includes three possible scenarios, mutually exclusive: progression of Dysmobility towards deeper stages, stabilization, and regression towards earlier stages.
- **Triaxial diagnosis**: Central part of the method for diagnosing Dysmobility. It includes the form of presentation, the time of evolution, and the staging of Dysmobility.
- **D-STAGING**: Hetero-applied system for continuum identification of stages of Disability in people aged 60 or over, with clinical, therapeutic, prognostic, and scientific objectives. It allows you to identify five stages of Dysmobility, with two substages each. That is, it consists of ten substages. It must be applied by personnel with competencies in geriatrics. Its application requires prior training.

Aging [2, 8]

- **Movement-Time (Theory)**: The theory of aging, which uses a new definition of aging based on the interactions between movement and time

- **Aging (definition)**: Product of the interaction between movement and time
- **Aging (formula)**: $E = M*t$ where 'E' is aging, 'M' is movement, and 't' is time)
- **Aging (7 characteristics)**:
  - Constant process that occurs in all elements, living and non-living (including ideas, philosophies, cultures, etc.).
  - Generates, in parallel, two effects: deterioration and maturation. There is no aging that is only deteriorative or only maturative. We live in a dynamic balance between both. In this way, 'deteriorating' aging is that which occurs due to 'deleterious', 'absent', and/or 'altered' movements; and 'healthy' (or 'maturational') aging is that which is achieved through 'protective' movements.
  - Inter- and transgenerational continuum: It does not begin or end; it just continues.
  - It is an original continuum: We all age in different ways.
  - It is an interpersonal continuum: The aging of one person influences the way others age. That is, we all age in complementary ways.
  - It is a multidimensional continuum: Biopsychosocial and spiritual, functional, cultural, architectural, artistic, etc.
  - It is a reversible continuum. We can influence some elements to limit or reverse deterioration or enhance maturation, producing healthy aging. Unfortunately, the opposite is also possible.

Health

- **Health (Definition 1)**: Study of the effects that movement has on the bodies that produce it (considering that body and movement are an indissoluble unit). Bodies suffer consequences of said movement, which go far beyond position changes in a spatial reference system.

– **Health (Definition 2)**: State of perfect mobility ('Eu-mobility').

References

1. Borel M, Vénizélos G. Chapters 2 and 3: Movement equations 1: location, kinematics and kinetics. Wiley; 2016.
2. Dinamarca J, Rubio R, Bonta C. Teoría de la Dismovilidad: Movimiento, tiempo y envejecimiento. In: En búsqueda de las bases de una única Teoría del Envejecimiento. Ediciones de la Fundación MAPFRE, premio Ayuda a la Investigación Ignacio de Larramendi 2007. Granada: Universidad de Granada; 2007. https://app.mapfre.com/ccm/content/documentos/fundacion/salud/becas/teoria-de-la-dismovilidad-movimientos-tiempo-y-envejecimiento.pdf.
3. Luis D-MJ. Chapter 33: Enfermedades musculoesqueléticas. In: d'Hyver C, Robledo LMG, Gil CHZ, editors. Geriatría. México City: Editorial El Manual Moderno; 2024.
4. Sennour Y, Counsell SR, Jones J, Weiner M. Development and implementation of a proactive geriatrics consultation model in collaboration with hospitalists. J Am Geriatr Soc. 2009;57(11):2139–45. https://doi.org/10.1111/j.1532-5415.2009.02496.x.
5. Inouye SK, Studenski S, Tinetti ME, Kuchel GA. Geriatric syndromes: clinical, research, and policy implications of a core geriatric concept. J Am Geriatr Soc. 2007;55(5):780–91. https://doi.org/10.1111/j.1532-5415.2007.01156.x.
6. Dinamarca-Montecinos JL. Dysmobility in geriatrics. A decade defining a clinical concept. Bol Hosp Vina del Mar 2012; 68(2):15–19
7. Dinamarca Montecinos JL. De la Inmovilidad a la Dismovilidad en Geriatría. Santiago: Ediciones de la Sociedad Chilena de Psicogeriatría; 2004.
8. Dinamarca-Montecinos JL. Teoría del Movimiento-Tiempo: Una nueva teoría para comprender el proceso de envejecer. Bol Hosp Viña del Mar. 2015;71(4):151–3.

Index

J. L. Dinamarca-Montecinos, *Dysmobility in Geriatrics*, https://doi.org/10.1007/978-3-031-72716-0

MIX
Papier aus verantwortungsvollen Quellen
Paper from responsible sources
FSC® C105338

If you have any concerns about our products, you can contact us on
ProductSafety@springernature.com

In case Publisher is established outside the EU, the EU authorized representative is:
Springer Nature Customer Service Center GmbH
Europaplatz 3, 69115 Heidelberg, Germany

Printed by Libri Plureos GmbH
in Hamburg, Germany